W9-ADS-852

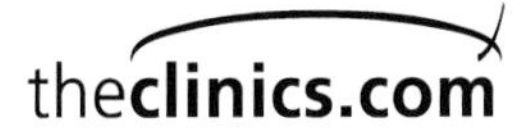

DENTAL CLINICS OF NORTH AMERICA

Handbook of Dental Practice

GUEST EDITORS
Harry Dym, DDS
Orrett E. Ogle, DDS

July 2008 • Volume 52 • Number 3

SAUNDERS

An Imprint of Elsevier, Inc.
PHILADELPHIA LONDON TORONTO MONTREAL SYDNEY TOKYO

W.B. SAUNDERS COMPANY
A Division of Elsevier Inc.

Elsevier Inc. • 1600 John F. Kennedy Boulevard • Suite 1800 • Philadelphia, Pennsylvania 19103-2899

http://www.dental.theclinics.com

DENTAL CLINICS OF NORTH AMERICA
July 2008
Editor: John Vassallo; j.vassallo@elsevier.com

Volume 52, Number 3
ISSN 0011-8532
ISBN-13: 978-1-4160-6285-1
ISBN-10: 1-4160-6285-8

Reprints: For copies of 100 or more, of articles in this publication, please contact the Commercial Reprints Department, Elsevier Inc., 360 Park Avenue South, New York, New York, 10010-1710. Tel.: (212) 633-3813, Fax: (212) 462-1935, E-mail: reprints@elsevier.com.

Dental Clinics of North America (ISSN 0011-8532) is published quarterly by Elsevier Inc., 360 Park Avenue South, New York, NY 10010-1710. Months of issue are January, April, July, and October. Business and Editorial Offices: 1600 John F. Kennedy Boulevard, Suite 1800, Philadelphia, PA 19103-2899. Customer Service Office: 6277 Sea Harbor Drive, Orlando, FL 32887-4800. Periodicals postage paid at New York, NY and additional mailing offices. Subscription prices are $188.00 per year (US individuals), $315.00 per year (US institutions), $91.00 per year (US students), $224.00 per year (Canadian individuals), $389.00 per year (Canadian institutions), $128.00 per year (Canadian students), $254.00 per year (international individuals), $389.00 per year (international institutions), and $128.00 per year (international students). International air speed delivery is included in all *Clinics* subscription prices. All prices are subject to change without notice. **POSTMASTER:** Send address changes to *Dental Clinics of North America*, Elsevier Periodicals Customer Service, 6277 Sea Harbor Drive, Orlando, FL 32887-4800. Customer Service: 1-800-654-2452 (US). From outside the United States, call 1-407-563-6020. Fax: 1-407-363-9661. E-mail: JournalsCustomerService-usa@elsevier.com.

The Dental Clinics of North America is covered in *MEDLINE/PubMed (Index Medicus), Current Contents/Clinical Medicine, ISI/BIOMED* and *Clinahl.*

Printed in the United States of America.

GUEST EDITORS

HARRY DYM, DDS, Chair, Department of Dentistry and Oral and Maxillofacial Surgery; and Director, Residency Training Program in Oral and Maxillofacial Surgery, The Brooklyn Hospital Center; Senior Attending, Woodhull Hospital, Brooklyn; Clinical Professor, Department of Oral and Maxillofacial Surgery, Columbia University College of Dental Medicine, New York, New York

ORRETT E. OGLE, DDS, Chief and Director, Residency Training Program in Oral and Maxillofacial Surgery, Department of Dentistry, Woodhull Hospital, Brooklyn; Assistant Clinical Professor, Oral and Maxillofacial Surgery, Columbia University, College of Dental Medicine, New York, New York

CONTRIBUTORS

SANJEEV BHATIA, DDS, FDS RCS(Eng), MDS, Chief Resident, Department of Oral and Maxillofacial Surgery, The Brooklyn Hospital Center, Brooklyn, New York

STANLEY BODNER, PhD, Senior P/T Faculty, Department of Social Science, Adelphi University-University College, Garden City; Private Practice Psychologist, Brooklyn, New York

RICARDO BOYCE, DDS, Program Director of General Dental Practice Residency Program, Department of Dentistry/Oral and Maxillofacial Surgery, The Brooklyn Hospital Center, Brooklyn; Part-time Clinical Professor, New York University College of Dentistry, New York, New York

LORI S. BRUELHEIDE, Department of Revenue Management, UK Healthcare; Formerly, Assistant Director for Clinical Operations, University of Kentucky, College of Dentistry, Kentucky Clinic Dentistry, Lexington, Kentucky

EARL CLARKSON, DDS, Director, Department of Oral and Maxillofacial Surgery, The Brooklyn Hospital Center, Brooklyn, New York

ERIC T.K. DEMANN, DMD, Assistant Professor, University of Kentucky, College of Dentistry, Kentucky Clinic Dentistry, Lexington, Kentucky

ROBERT J. DIECIDUE, DMD, MD, MBA, MSPH, Department of Oral and Maxillofacial Surgery, Thomas Jefferson University Hospital, Philadelphia, Pennsylvania

HARRY DYM, DDS, Chair, Department of Dentistry and Oral and Maxillofacial Surgery; and Director, Residency Training Program in Oral and Maxillofacial Surgery, The Brooklyn Hospital Center; Senior Attending, Woodhull Hospital, Brooklyn; Clinical Professor, Department of Oral and Maxillofacial Surgery, Columbia University College of Dental Medicine, New York, New York

ROBERT Q. FRAZER, DDS, Assistant Professor, Division of Prosthodontics, University of Kentucky, College of Dentistry, Lexington, Kentucky

RICHARD H. HAUG, DDS, Professor of Oral and Maxillofacial Surgery, and Executive Associate Dean, University of Kentucky, College of Dentistry, Lexington, Kentucky

GLENA JARBOE, Dental Quality Assurance Manager, University of Kentucky, College of Dentistry, Lexington, Kentucky

CHRISTINE LEVITT, Administrative Staff Officer III, Office of Administrative Affairs, University of Kentucky, College of Dentistry, Lexington, Kentucky

PHILLIP MCIVER, DDS, Department of Oral and Maxillofacial Surgery, Harlem Hospital Center, New York, New York

JUSTIN MULL, DMD, Chief Resident of Oral and Maxillofacial Surgery, Department of Dentistry/Oral and Maxillofacial Surgery, The Brooklyn Hospital Center, Brooklyn, New York

REBECCA H. NAPIER, Associate Administrative Director, Department of Surgery; and Formerly, Clinical Unit Manager for Oral and Maxillofacial Surgery, University of Kentucky, College of Dentistry, Lexington, Kentucky

IAN M. NELSON, CPA, LLC, Sole Practitioner, West Orange, New Jersey

ORRETT E. OGLE, DDS, Chief and Director, Residency Training Program in Oral and Maxillofacial Surgery, Department of Dentistry, Woodhull Hospital, Brooklyn; Assistant Clinical Professor, Oral and Maxillofacial Surgery, Columbia University, College of Dental Medicine, New York, New York

ORVILLE PALMER, MD, MPH, FRCSC, Division of Otolaryngology, Head and Neck Surgery, Department of Surgery, Harlem Hospital Center; Department of Otolaryngology, Columbia University College of Physicians and Surgeons, New York, New York

KEITH E. SHELTON, MPA, Assistant Dean for Clinical Administration, University of Kentucky, College of Dentistry, Lexington, Kentucky

PAMELA S. STEIN, DMD, Assistant Professor of Anatomy and Neurobiology, University of Kentucky, College of Medicine, Lexington, Kentucky

KENNETH C. THOMALLA, CPA, CLU, CFPR, Treloar and Heisel, Inc., Orland Park, Illinois

MARK V. THOMAS, DMD, Associate Professor and Chief of Periodontology, Division of Periodontology, University of Kentucky, College of Dentistry, Lexington, Kentucky

JEFFREY WHERRY, CLU, CFPR, New Castle, Pennsylvania

EDMUND WUN, DDS, Department of Oral and Maxillofacial Surgery, The Brooklyn Hospital Center, Brooklyn, New York

CONTENTS

FORTHCOMING ISSUES

October 2008

Contemporary Dental and Maxillofacial Imaging
Steven L. Thomas, DDS, MS
and Christos Angelopoulos, DDS, MS, *Guest Editors*

January 2009

Evidence-Based Dentistry
Mark V. Thomas, DMD, *Guest Editor*

April 2009

Special Care Dentistry
Burton S. Wasserman, DDS, *Guest Editor*

RECENT ISSUES

April 2008

Dental Public Health
Oscar Arevalo, DDS, ScD, MBS, MS
and Amit Chattopadhyay, PhD, MPH, MDS, BDS (Hons),
Guest Editors

January 2008

Management of the Oncologic Patient
Sook-Bin Woo, DMD, MMSc and
Nathaniel S. Treister, DMD, DMSc, *Guest Editors*

October 2007

Dentistry's Role in Disaster Response
Michael D. Colvard, DDS, MTS, MS, *Guest Editor*

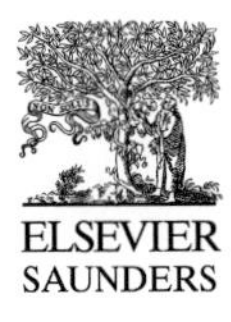

Dent Clin N Am 52 (2008) xiii

THE DENTAL CLINICS OF NORTH AMERICA

Dedication

This issue is dedicated to Mr. Chaim Dym, a quiet and humble man possessed of great spiritual strength who continues to be a moral and ethical beacon for his children, grandchildren, and great-grandchildren. This issue also is dedicated to Mrs. Hedy Rosner, a woman of valor who has lived a life dedicated to her children, grandchildren, and great-grandchildren.

Harry Dym, DDS

doi:10.1016/j.cden.2008.04.002

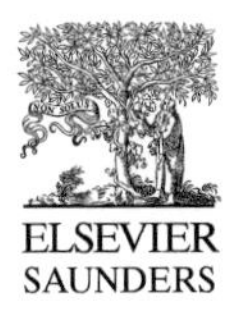

THE DENTAL CLINICS OF NORTH AMERICA

Dent Clin N Am 52 (2008) xv–xvii

Preface

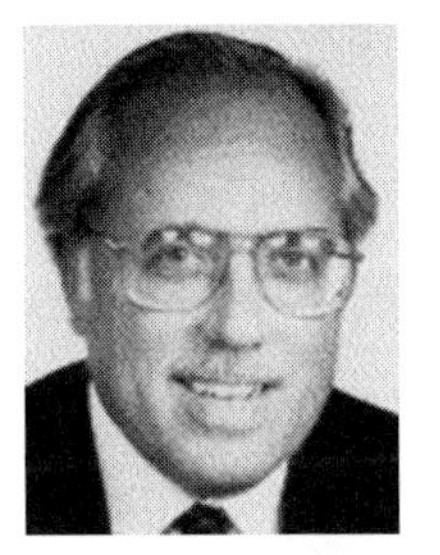

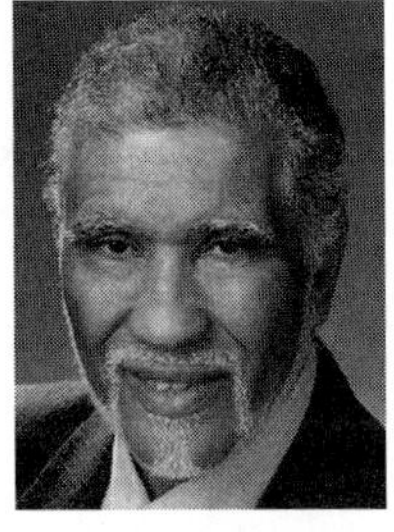

Harry Dym, DDS Orrett E. Ogle, DDS
Guest Editors

"It is not the years in your life, but the life in your years that counts"
Adlai Stevenson

Today's dental graduates are entering the work environment with a greater clinical knowledge base than ever before. The amount of scientific information necessary for the current general dentist who wishes to practice the full scope of comprehensive general dentistry is staggering and forever increasing, and the level of technical skills awareness of new product information required also is increasing. Given the previously stated remarks, it often seems that other areas of knowledge that are almost as important to developing a successful clinical practice are sometimes overlooked or given short shrift by general dentists and dental specialists alike. The goal of this issue, entitled "Handbook of Dental Practice", is to gather vital practice information (other than direct clinical information) that all recent dental graduates and even senior dentists working in private practice need to be aware of to effectively manage a busy modern day dental practice.

We are grateful to our contributors who, despite their busy work schedules, were able to contribute to this issue. They fulfilled our goals and

Dr. Ogle's picture by Patrick Ashley.

0011-8532/08/$ - see front matter
doi:10.1016/j.cden.2008.04.001

objectives and completed their mission successfully. We hope the readership finds this issue helpful and useful as a reference guide as they strive to deliver quality dental care in an ever changing and challenging healthcare environment.

This issue marks our eighth issue serving as guest editors for the *Clinics of North America* series (*Dental Clinics of North America* and *Oral and Maxillofacial Surgery Clinics of North America*), and we acknowledge Elsevier for its contributions to the dental profession. We also thank our excellent editor, John Vassallo, for his capable assistance and friendship.

On a personal note, Dr. Dym acknowledges Mr. Jonathan M. Weld and Mr. Carlos Naudon (Chair and Vice Chair of the Brooklyn Hospital Board of Trustees), Mr. Samuel Lehrfeld (President and CEO of The Brooklyn Hospital Center), Mr. Paul Albertson (Executive Vice President and Chief Operating Officer), and Dr. John Carroll (Chief Medical Officer of The Brooklyn Hospital Center) for their strong commitment to dentistry and oral and maxillofacial surgery and their guidance and friendship for the past 5 years. Mr. George Harris, a dedicated member of the Board of Trustees at The Brooklyn Hospital Center and the Lucius Littauer Foundation, has been a long time supporter of the Dental/Oral and Maxilliofacial Surgery residency programs at our hospital, and he has my (Dr. Dym) profound gratitude and respect.

I (Dr. Dym) specially mention Dr. Earl Clarkson and my co-guest editor, Dr. Orrett Ogle, with whom I have had the pleasure and honor to work side by side with in resident education for over a quarter of a century; they are truly extraordinary teachers and represent the best in our profession. I (Dr. Dym) also appreciate the contributions of my Executive Administrative Assistant, Felipe DeJesus, for his dedicated service to our Dental/Oral and Maxilliofacial Surgery department.

I (Dr. Dym) also thank my mentor of almost 3 decades, Dr. Peter M. Sherman (Chairman of Dentistry and Oral and Maxillofacial Surgery at Woodhull Medical Center), who taught me that "the best reward for a job well done is a job well done". I say thank you for these many years of friendship.

I (Dr. Dym) thank my wife (Friedy), my children (Yehoshua, Chani, Hindy, Daniel, Michal and Akiva), and my grandchildren (Noah and Malka) for adding the life to my years.

Harry Dym, DDS
Director, Residency Training Program in
Oral and Maxillofacial Surgery
Department of Dentistry and Oral Maxillofacial Surgery
The Brooklyn Hospital Center
121 Dekalb Avenue
Brooklyn, NY 11201, USA

E-mail address: hdymdds@yahoo.com

Orrett E. Ogle, DDS
Chief and Director
Residency Training Program in
Oral and Maxillofacial Surgery
Department of Dentistry
Woodhull Hospital
760 Broadway
Brooklyn, NY 11206, USA

E-mail address: orrett.ogle@woodhullhc.nychhc.org

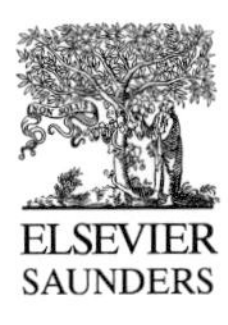

ELSEVIER
SAUNDERS

Dent Clin N Am 52 (2008) 469–481

THE DENTAL CLINICS OF NORTH AMERICA

Credentialing

Orrett E. Ogle, DDS[a,b,*]

[a]*Department of Dentistry, Woodhull Hospital, 760 Broadway, Brooklyn, NY 11206, USA*
[b]*Columbia University, College of Dental Medicine, 630 West 168th Street, New York, NY 10032, USA*

Credentialing is the administrative process for validating the qualifications of licensed professionals and appraising their background. The process generally involves an objective evaluation of a subject's current licensure, training or experience, competence, and ability to provide particular services or perform particular procedures. It is used by hospitals and other health care facilities, educational institutions, and insurance companies to ensure the qualification of their clinicians and to grant privileges to provide specific services and perform different medical or dental procedures. The process is also used by state dental boards to grant licensure or to decide on whether to accept candidates from other states or jurisdictions for licensure by qualifications only. This article familiarizes the reader with the credentialing process and reviews documentation that is needed to be credentialed by certain organizations.

Standard credentialing information that generally is required after graduation from dental school includes the following:

- Biographic information
- Dental practice information
- Current state dental license
- Current Drug Enforcement Administration (DEA) certificate
- Current state controlled substance certification
- Malpractice coverage summary
- Specialty verification
- Board eligibility or certification verification
- National Practitioner Data Bank (NPDB) report

* Corresponding author. Department of Dentistry/Oral and Maxillofacial Surgery, Woodhull Medical and Mental Health Center, 760 Broadway, Brooklyn, NY 11206-5317.
E-mail address: orrett.ogle@woodhullhc.nychhc.org

0011-8532/08/$ - see front matter
doi:10.1016/j.cden.2008.02.001 ***dental.theclinics.com***

The credentialing process involves initial data gathering, primary source verification, and enhanced data gathering and verification.

Initial data gathering

Initial data gathering is the process of securing a complete application with demographic information and professional credentials. It may be done by an individual institution or a network, the credentialing or peer review department of an insurance company, a professional credentialing specialist, or a regional electronic service. All questions on the credentialing application must be answered. Failure to answer all questions or to provide all requested documentation would force the credentialing committee to withdraw the dentist's application. Similarly, information provided by the dentist must be held in the strictest confidence.

Primary source verification

Primary source verification is the process of authenticating information provided by the dentist during the initial data gathering. Dentists practicing within a community must comply with all applicable local, state, and federal laws and regulations. This compliance will vary by states or territories and, in addition to state license, may include matters related to disease and infection control, child abuse and domestic violence, infected waste material, and so on. Hospitals also have specific and unique requirements for practicing within their confines. Credentialing committees verify compliance with the necessary regulations for their region and organization. Some of the verification may be done by direct interaction with sources such as state dental boards and the NPDB via secure Internet and digital technologies or by the dentist providing proof such as malpractice certification, basis life support (BLS) or advanced cardiac life support (ACLS) cards, and proof of taking an infection control course. Primary source verification includes all or several of the items discussed in the following sections.

State licensure

A photocopy of a current state dental license (with the license number and issue date) is always requested. This copy is kept on file along with proof of current registration. The credentialing committee or department will validate that the dentist's license to practice is active and unencumbered and will confirm whether there are any sanctions against the license. This information can be obtained directly from individual state licensing boards of dentistry.

National practitioner data bank query

The NPDB is a clearinghouse of information relating to medical malpractice payments and adverse actions taken against physicians, dentists, and other licensed health care practitioners in regards to restrictions or limitations of clinical privileges and sanctions by professional associations. Hospitals and other health care entities, including professional societies and state licensing boards, use the information contained in the NPDB in conjunction with information from other sources when granting clinical privileges or in employment, affiliation, or licensure decisions.

The information on the professional competence and conduct of physicians and dentists that is provided by the NPDB is only available to state licensing boards, hospitals and other health care entities, professional societies, certain federal agencies, and other entities specifically named under section 11134(b) of The Health Care Quality Improvement Act of 1986. Hospitals are the only health care entity with federal mandatory requirements for querying the NPDB. Information is not available to the general public, and practitioners may query the NPDB regarding themselves at any time. Several commercial dental insurance companies state on their Web page that they use information from the NPDB when considering participation on their provider panels. Health maintenance organizations (HMOs) that are entering into an affiliation relationship with a dentist who has applied for affiliation may access the information [1] and are mandated to do so in certain localities.

The purpose of the NPDB is to improve the quality of health care by encouraging state licensing boards, hospitals and other health care entities (including insurance companies), and professional societies to identify and discipline persons who engage in unprofessional behavior and to restrict the ability of incompetent physicians, dentists, and other health care practitioners to move from state to state without disclosure or discovery of previous medical malpractice payment and adverse action history. Adverse actions can involve licensure, denial or withdrawal of clinical privileges, expulsion from membership in a professional society, and exclusions from Medicare and Medicaid.

National technical information service

A photocopy of a current DEA certificate will be requested. Validation of the practitioner's license to prescribe drugs is done through the National Technical Information Service (NTIS). The NTIS is an agency in the Technology Administration of the US Department of Commerce that serves as the US government repository for results of research and development and for other information produced by and for the government as well as a variety of public and private sources. One of the products available from the NTIS is the complete official DEA database of persons and organizations certified to prescribe or handle controlled substances under the Controlled Substances Act. The DEA authorizes the use of this database and the inclusion of any individual or organization in the database as proof of that entity's registration with the DEA.

General anesthesia permit (if applicable)

Validation of the practitioner's permit to administer anesthesia is required. A photocopy of the certification for general anesthesia or conscious sedation permit is required if the applicant wishes to use sedation within a hospital or bill for sedation in a private office. Most states require additional permits or licenses for dentists who are trained in the administration of substances that produce general anesthesia, deep sedation, or conscious sedation, or for nitrous oxide sedation in patients being treated by the licensee, although most states omit nitrous oxide. The American Dental Association (ADA) position statement on the use of conscious sedation, deep sedation, and general anesthesia in dentistry advocates that state dental boards have a responsibility to ensure that only dentists who are properly trained, experienced, and competent are allowed to use conscious sedation, deep sedation, and general anesthesia within their jurisdictions [2].

Malpractice insurance

Current active malpractice coverage is one of the credentialing standards set by nearly all nongovernmental organizations and dental insurance companies, and this information is routinely collected as part of the process. This verification usually requires a photocopy of the current malpractice insurance certificate (with the policy number, levels of individual aggregate coverage, and dates of coverage) or a verification from the insurance carrier itself. Most organizations want an assurance that the dentist carries adequate malpractice insurance, usually $1,000,000 per occurrence and $3,000,000 per aggregate.

Specialty certification

To obtain a specialty license, to practice as a specialist within a hospital or an academic institution, or to bill an insurance carrier as a specialist, proof of specialty training is required. To become a specialist, one must be trained in a residency or advanced graduate training program accredited by the ADA. Once the residency is completed, the doctor is granted a certificate of specialty training. Many specialty programs require advanced degrees such as MD (specific to oral and maxillofacial surgery), MS, or PhD.

There are nine recognized dental specialties in the United States [3]: dental public health, endodontics, oral and maxillofacial pathology, oral and maxillofacial radiology, oral and maxillofacial surgery, orthodontics and dentofacial orthopedics, pediatric dentistry, periodontics, and prosthodontics.

Dentists who receive formal education in these fields are designated as being "board eligible" and can advertise exclusive titles such as orthodontist, oral and maxillofacial surgeon, endodontist, pedodontist, periodontist, or prosthodontist and are educationally eligible to sit examinations to become "board certified." Many insurance companies require board certification after a specific time to remain listed as a specialist on their panels. Hospitals also require board certification.

The specialist designations are registrable titles and in the United States are controlled by the ADA. The Dental Practice Act of most states forbids a licensed and registered dentist to designate in any manner that he or she has limited their practice to one of the specialty areas of dentistry expressly approved by the ADA unless such dentist has completed the required advanced or postgraduate education in the area of such specialty. Some states issue a specialty license or require notification of the state's dental commission of such limitation of practice. Pseudo-specialists such as a cosmetic dentist, dental implantologist, or temporomandibular joint specialist are not fields that people are generally credentialed in as a specialist, and there are restrictions on allowing these dentists to call themselves specialists in these fields in certain jurisdictions and by some local dental associations. General practitioners can provide services in specialty areas such as oral surgery, endodontics, or periodontics, but they cannot bill as a specialist and may not receive reimbursement at the specialist fees.

Medicaid

Dental Medicaid is fairly limited, and the number of dentists participating in the program is decreasing. Some private insurance carriers, HMOs, and hospitals may try to determine whether sanctions have been imposed on the practitioner by the federal government's Office of Inspector General or Office of Personnel Management. Exclusion for cause by Medicaid may be used by an insurance company to deny an applicant participation on their closed panel.

Enhanced data gathering

Enhanced data gathering involves research and collection of additional information concerning issues such as criminal convictions, sexual misconduct allegations or investigations, child abuse allegations or investigations, health issues and substance abuse, unprofessional conduct, and inappropriate prescribing practices.

Some of this enhanced data gathering is normally collected by a "yes/no" form on which the applicant is required to sign an affidavit. "Yes" responses require a written detailed explanation. Some jurisdictions will require the applicant to obtain a report from the Criminal Justice Information Services (CJIS) division of the FBI.

The CJIS is a computerized criminal justice information system within the FBI that provides timely and relevant criminal justice information concerning individuals to qualified law enforcement bodies as well as civilians and academic, employment, and licensing agencies. The database of the

CJIS is, for the most part, supplied to the FBI on a monthly basis by federal, state, and local law enforcement agencies. The FBI assembles the data and distributes it to law enforcement organizations and civilian entities interested in this information. To obtain the identification record, each applicant must submit in writing to the FBI [CJIS Division, ATTN: SCU, Mod. D-2, 1000 Custer Hollow Road, Clarksburg, WV 26306, phone (304) 625-3878] a signed letter stating the reason for requesting the identification record (licensure application), a completed fingerprint card, and a certified check or money order for $18.00 (2007) made payable to the Treasure of the United States. The fingerprint form may be downloaded from the FBI Web site at http://www.fbi.gov/hq/cjisd/pdf/fpcardb.pdf.

Other information can be obtained from the Division of Professional Conduct of each state.

Credentialing by specific organizations

State board of dentistry

A state board of dentistry will most likely be the first to credential a dentist for the purpose of granting a license to practice dentistry. The qualifications to obtain a dental license in a particular state are controlled by the Dental Practice Act of the individual state. Documentation required by all 50 states includes the following:

- A written application for a license must be signed by the applicant.
- Proof of age of at least 21 years and of good moral character must be provided.
- A diploma from a dental college accredited by the ADA conferring a dental degree (DDS or DMD) must be provided.
- Successful completion of an examination authorized or given by the state board in the theory and practice of the science of dentistry must be achieved. All 50 states recognize the certificate granted by the National Board of Dental Examiners; however, passing scores may be established by the individual state boards.
- Successful completion of a clinical examination conducted by the state dental board of examiners or by an approved regional testing service in lieu of the state examination must be achieved. Successful completion means that the applicant has achieved a minimum passing score on the regional examinations as determined by the regional testing service. New York State now requires the successful completion of a 1 year general practice residency.
- Payment of a fee is required.

Other items that may be required are an infection control course certification, documentation of having attended a child abuse recognition course, a BLS certificate, and a jurisprudence test.

Relicensure

Dentists are re-credentialed for renewal of their license every 2 or 3 years as mandated by their state. This process usually involves an update in biographic data, criminal convictions, sexual misconduct, substance abuse, the suspension by state professional associations, unprofessional conduct, DEA violations, and current infection control and child abuse certificates. This data gathering is collected by a "yes/no" form on which the applicant is required to sign an affidavit. "Yes" responses require a written detailed explanation.

Mandatory continuing education (CE) is an almost universal requirement for relicensure of dentists in the United States. A survey in 2005 found that 45 states and the District of Columbia mandated CE for relicensure [4]. The number of hours, period of time, and the types of CE vary by state. Some state dental boards have made distinctions about the acceptability of CE credits. For instance, some state dental boards set minimums, maximums, or both for clinical and nonclinical credit hours. Others require a minimum number of credit hours on certain subjects, such as infection control, child abuse, HIV/AIDS, and BLS. Another categorization divides CE credits into those earned through independent study and on-site courses [4].

Reporting of CE credits earned over the mandated time span is most often done by an affidavit indicating that the applicant has completed the required minimum number of hours of CE in approved courses as required by the state. The affidavit rarely requires a listing of courses. The affidavit is considered to be prima facie evidence that the applicant has obtained the minimum number of required CE hours in approved courses. In these cases, verification is done by random audits. Another method of recording CE credits is through a state agency or an organization such as the state dental society or the Academy of General Dentistry. Clinicians should keep their own log of courses taken along with the documentation of attendance.

Licensure by credentials (also known as licensure by recognition)

Licensure by recognition is a process by which a state board of dentistry grants a dental license to an individual based on its determination that the candidate has previously met requirements for initial licensure in another jurisdiction, holds a current state license to practice in another state of the United States, and has practiced for a minimum specified amount of time before application (usually 5 years) in a state that has licensure standards equivalent to the one where licensure by credentials is being sought. If the candidate meets all of the required criteria, a license is granted upon payment of the fee. The purpose of this credentialing is to prevent dentists who are inept, addicted to drugs, or convicted of a crime from going state-to-state undetected.

Unlike in medicine, dentistry does not have a national credentialing system that would allow dentists to practice in any US state; therefore, dentists must go through a system of state-by-state licensure. Although the process of obtaining a license by credentialing varies by state, common documents that may be requested are as follows:

- Some state boards may require a report from all states or territories of the United States or District of Columbia where the applicant has ever held or currently holds a dental license to verify a current active license. The license must be "active" (not under suspension), and there should be no sanctions against the license. Reasons for surrendering a license may be requested.
- Continuing dental education credits that meet the requirements for the state to which the candidate is applying will need to be provided. The applicant will need to submit the certification of attendance.
- A letter attesting to the "good character" of the applicant from the state dental society or association may need to be provided.
- The applicant may need to pass a written jurisprudence examination on the Dental Practice Act of the state.
- Proof of successfully passing the dental National Boards I and II, administered by the Council of National Board of Dental Examiners, must be provided.
- The applicant may be asked to personally appear before the credentialing committee of the board for an interview.
- A search for a criminal background record may be performed.
- A review of the applicant's practice history may be requested.

Insurance panels

Private insurance carriers assemble a panel of participating dentists who agree to accept the fees established by the insurance companies. Because these agreements are dictated by the insurance companies, "business criteria" become a part of the credentialing process, and the payee will first verify whether the provider falls within their business criteria for network participation.

The credentialing process of HMOs, unions, and other insurance companies is intended to evaluate the qualifications of dentists who provide care to their members but often becomes a process designed to find dentists that meet the requirements necessary to be a participating provider. With more reputable insurance companies, the process will involve the data gathering and verification steps discussed previously. The following is a checklist of documents that are needed when an application is made to participate on an insurance panel:

- A photocopy must be provided of the current state dental license (with the license number, issue date, and expiration date). This information is verified with the state dental board.

- A photocopy must be provided of a current DEA certificate. The dentist must be able to prescribe medications, specifically antibiotics and analgesics.
- A photocopy must be provided of the current malpractice insurance certificate (with the policy number, levels of individual aggregate coverage, and dates of coverage). This certificate is one of the credentialing standards set by nearly all dental insurers, and this information is routinely collected as part of the process. The insurers want to guarantee their members that the dentists who participate in their programs carry adequate malpractice insurance.
- A photocopy must be provided of specialty certifications or general anesthesia or conscious sedation permits, if applicable.

Some of the more selective health insurance companies will query the NPDB before accepting applicants to their panel, and they can (and some will) conduct peer and performance reviews of existing participating practitioners. Because participating dentists are independent practitioners in private or group practice and are neither agents nor employees of insurance companies or HMOs, their credentialing process cannot guarantee any level of quality or the type of service provided to their members by the participating dentists.

Hospital staff membership

The process of applying for and obtaining hospital privileges can be long and arduous and is the most involved credentialing process that a dentist will undergo. This process is somewhat similar to what has been mentioned previously. The applicant will need to fill out a biographic form that often includes details of clinical experience such as residency or internships, previous hospital privileges, any previous denial, suspension, or revocation of privileges, and any involvement in malpractice suits or college investigations. Additional items that are often requested are a resume, ACLS and advanced trauma life support certificates, evidence of successful completion of clinical procedures relevant to clinical practice, reference letters, and a recent photograph.

The Joint Commission on Accreditation of Healthcare Organizations (JCAHO) specifies four core criteria that should be met when credentialing licensed independent practitioners: (1) current licensure, (2) relevant training or experience, (3) current competence (defined as letters from authoritative sources attesting to the applicant's scope and level of performance), and (4) the ability to perform privileges requested.

The terms *credentials* and *privileges* define separate entities that are determined independently, and appropriate documentation will be required for each. The credentialing criteria for appointment to the medical staff are the general requirements that must be met by all applicants for medical staff appointment and by all medical professionals currently practicing in the hospital. The criteria for delineation of clinical privileges, on the other hand, specify the certification or specific training and experience needed to be eligible for specific clinical privileges. The ruling body that accredits hospitals—the JCAHO—requires that "All individuals who are permitted by law and by the hospital to provide patient care services independently in the hospital have delineated clinical privileges." For clinical privileges, documentation will be required to determine competence, relevant education, training, and experience with respect to the particular procedures that he or she seeks to perform.

It is the duty of the hospital and its medical staff office to ensure that the physicians (the term *physician* also includes dentists) on staff are qualified and competent to deliver care. A primary purpose is not only to evaluate the qualifications of the physician but also to determine the clinical competence, experience, and judgment of that physician. Because one of the main purposes of credentialing in the hospital is to ensure a high quality of care, competency becomes an important factor. Granting hospital privileges to a physician or dentist with inadequate clinical qualifications will obviously have important patient care and legal implications. In the current litigious climate, hospitals have implemented stringent privileging processes to protect against malpractice suits. The medical staff office of the hospital must determine whether the applicant for privileges has the training and experience needed to ensure competence in the procedures in which he or she is seeking privileges and must translate the information gained into an appropriate course of action (ie, to grant or deny privileges).

Like their medical counterparts, dentists wishing to provide patient care in the hospital must seek delineation of their clinical privileges. Delineation is the process by which the hospital determines what specific procedures may be performed by each medical staff applicant and appointee in the hospital. The criteria for granting clinical privileges are outlined in the medical staff bylaws and differ between institutions. Clinical privileges granted to a dentist must be consistent with all applicable state laws and regulations, and the services provided must be within the scope of practice. This criterion has presented some difficulties to oral and maxillofacial surgeons who do not have a medical license and who seek privileges to provide an expanded scope of care. Hospitals that grant privileges to a dentist will first verify that the individual is properly licensed (dental, medical, or both [ie, a double-degree oral surgeon]) and is currently registered by the state. They will also query the NPDB and all of the other agencies previously mentioned before granting privileges.

Privilege and competency

The term *clinical privilege* defines an authorization granted to a practitioner by a local institution to perform a particular procedure or clinical service within the confines of the institution and is among the stickiest of all credentialing issues. The clinician must show that his or her training and experience qualifies him or her for the privileges being requested. A formal process for delineating privileges will be spelled out by the medical staff and departmental bylaws, policies, rules, or regulations, as well as by a program of peer review that evaluates the clinical performance on reappointments. The JCAHO accreditation manual specifically indicates that one of the responsibilities of a departmental chairperson or a chief of division is "recommending to the medical staff the criteria for clinical privileges in the department."

The term *competence* is used to define a standardized requirement for an individual to properly perform a specific task. It is the skill set that is essential for a dentist to begin independent unsupervised dental practice. Competency includes knowledge, experience, critical thinking and problem-solving skills, and technical and procedural skills that become an integral whole during the rendering of patient care [5].

In 1997 the American Dental Educators Association (formerly The American Association of Dental Schools) issued a document containing 63 competency statements [6] that have been used by dental schools as the educational goal of the predoctoral curriculum in the United States. The competency statements standardize expected learning outcomes and are the tool used by the curriculum developers and content experts of each dental school to select instructional strategies, provide relevancy of context, and ensure the most relevant and up to date dental content for their 4-year DDS/DMD curriculum that will result in the expected learning outcomes. The Committee on Dental Accreditation monitors each dental school for the quality of their educational standards. All dentists who graduate from an ADA-accredited dental school and who are licensed by a state will possess competency in certain basic clinical skills and diagnostic knowledge. These basic competencies can be used throughout the United States for granting privileges.

Hospital administrators and the JCAHO have considered the delineation of privileges to be the ultimate in establishing and guaranteeing high standards for patient care. To maintain this "guarantee" and to protect themselves from malpractice suits, hospitals have turned to core privileging. The core privileging approach uses predefined criteria established by the medical staff association and the departmental chairperson to set minimum standards of clinical activities that any appropriately trained and licensed practitioner would be competent to perform and then verifies the qualifications of the applicant against these criteria. Core privileges cover the range of clinical expertise gained through dental school education, training (residency and other postgraduate activity), and ongoing clinical practice. These skills endure throughout an active professional career. These criteria apply to a specialty or procedure and not to a specific department. They should allow for all qualified physicians to perform a basic procedure or treatment for which they are trained and should take away the "turf war." To gain more extensive privileges (referred to as special privileges), the applicant must prove evidence of education, training, and experience, and demonstrated current competence, ability, and judgment. Special privileges refer to certain operative or invasive procedures and clinical conditions for which training or expertise is not expected to have been achieved in dental school or, in general, is not routinely offered in the DDS/DMD curriculum or in every residency program. For special privileges, it is often expected that one must perform a minimum number of procedures each year to maintain clinical competency.

Credentialing problems

What happens if your request for privileges has been denied or restricted? The JCAHO stipulates that there must be an appeal process; however, this process may be long, because medical credential committees may only meet annually, biannually, or quarterly, and sometimes documents may have to go through more than one committee. The applicant should ensure that the specific information regarding the decision is obtained in writing, and that the letter explicitly states the reasons why privileges have been denied or restricted. If there are questions regarding training or documentation, the applicant should find out from the department chairperson under what circumstances these privileges may be obtained. Are there reasons other than those that have been stated in writing, such as other practitioners and not enough patients or questions regarding the scope of practice? Were privileges for cosmetic surgery denied because the applicant was a dentist? The applicant should keep written notes on any conversations related to his or her attempts to obtain privileges. Try to work with the department chairperson before seeking legal channels. A legal challenge should be the last resort.

If denial seems inevitable, it may be in one's best interest to remove an application from consideration before a negative vote. Managed care applications or future hospital staff applications may ask, "Have you ever been denied hospital privileges?" Answering "yes" may indicate that there is a problem with your credentials or a worse situation, that is, you were trying to obtain privileges for procedures that you were not qualified to perform. This discovery would harm the dentist's credibility with further hospital applications and may even end up in the NPDB. A withdrawn application may be resubmitted with more documentation to demonstrate that the dentist's training and experience qualify him or her for the privileges requested.

Summary

Credentialing is the method of ensuring professional qualification and competency. It demonstrates that one is qualified to practice dentistry independently and, in the hospital setting, that one is competent to perform requested procedures. Credentialing usually requires documentation of proof of graduation, state licenses, malpractice insurance, completion of CE requirements, and professional experience, and a curriculum vitae and other similar documentation. It is wise to gather these documents before beginning the process and to always have updated copies. In this article, an attempt was made to familiarize the reader with some of the intricacies of the process, particularly the method of gaining hospital privileges.

References

[1] Title IV of Public Law 99-660. The Health Care Quality Improvement Act of 1986, 42 USC §11137 (01/26/98), Chapter 117, Subchapter II, Reporting of Information §11137. (a) Miscellaneous provisions.
[2] ADA position and statements: use of conscious sedation, deep sedation and general anesthesia in dentistry. Available at: http://www.ada.org/prof/resources/positions/statements/useof.asp#state. Accessed July 2007.
[3] ADA recognized dental specialties. Available at: www.ada.org/prof/ed/specialties/specialty_certifying_report.pdf. Accessed July 2007.
[4] Schleyer TK, Dodell D. Continuing dental education requirements for relicensure in the United States. J Am Dent Assoc 2005;136(10):1450–6.
[5] American Dental Educators Association (ADEA). Call for comments: competencies for the new general dentist. Letter to ADEA members and dental education communities of interest, July 16, 2007.
[6] Exhibit 6: competencies for the new dentist (as approved by the 1997 House of Delegates). J Dent Educ 2004;68(7):742–4.

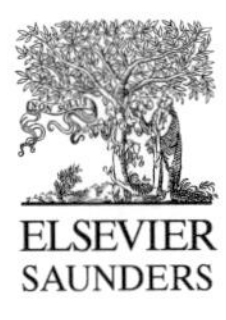
ELSEVIER
SAUNDERS

THE DENTAL CLINICS OF NORTH AMERICA

Dent Clin N Am 52 (2008) 483–493

Evaluating a Dental Practice for Purchase or Associateship

Robert J. Diecidue, DMD, MD, MBA, MSPH

Department of Oral and Maxillofacial Surgery, Thomas Jefferson University Hospital, Philadelphia, PA, USA

The decision to set up an independent practice or become an associate in an existing practice is one that every dentist faces at some point. Each decision is unique, balanced by individual professional goals and personal needs, and is generally based on multiple considerations. Although this fork in the road is not easy to navigate, it can be successful and very fulfilling if accompanied by adequate preparation, methodical progress, and support of appropriate professional advisors or consultants. The goal of this article is to review the various factors that should be considered, particularly evaluation of a dental practice for purchase or associateship.

General considerations

The decision about where and how to practice can affect a dentist's life. Reviewing personal and professional needs and goals is an important first step. Dentists must decide where they want to practice, what type of practice is appropriate for their personality, and what fits their current life situation and future life goals. Once these issues have been clarified, dentists should review staff and operating privileges, and available resources for continuing education in the preferred geographic area. These criteria are important in establishing and sustaining any new practice, and critical to professional development.

Another basic issue to consider is whether ownership or associateship would be appropriate. Although both require investing time and energy in research and preparation before proceeding, each may be appropriate for different reasons and circumstances, based largely on personality, comfort level, and overall goals. If ownership is preferred, the option of setting up

E-mail address: diecidue@jeffersonhospital.org

doi:10.1016/j.cden.2008.03.001 **dental.theclinics.com**

a brand new practice should be weighed against buying an established practice. Both options are available for anyone wanting to establish a solo practice.

Purchasing an established practice is a good option if the right practice can be found in the preferred geographic area. However some pros and cons must be considered.

In an established practice, people and systems are already in place and a referral base and an experienced and trained staff are available. These factors can assure a shorter time to begin operating the new practice. However, the condition of existing equipment and furniture must be determined and the cost of any refurbishment incorporated in the assessment. Furthermore, the need for a transition process for the practice, staff, and patients and the sensitivities involved must be considered to assure a successful conversion from the previous ownership and establish one's position in the new practice. Management professionals and transition coaches can assist and offer guidance in this process.

If opening a new practice is preferred, then research on the demographics and dental needs in the new area, the cost of purchasing a new site or repurposing an existing one, hiring of new staff, and establishing vendor relations are additional responsibilities that should be considered.

However, if an associateship is the initial choice, current opportunities and future options must be considered, such as an option to buy, which may be important in the longer term. Regardless of the choice, all licensing requirements must be researched and compliance guaranteed.

Once the decision is made, multiple practices should be evaluated before the choice is finalized. Creating an advisory team may be worthwhile to help guide the initial decision-making process and subsequent establishment and ongoing management. Table 1 provides a list of professionals that can assist in the valuation of a practice and assure that appropriate professional advice and guidance are obtained for various legal, financial, or management issues.

Valuation: establishing and evaluating the economic aspects of a practice

The *Guide for Dentists* published by the American Dental Association (ADA) notes that a dental practice's value should be viewed as fair market value (FMV) [1]. FMV may be defined as the cash or cash-equivalent value of a viable operating identity (ie, the practice) and is the most likely price on which a typical and rational buyer and seller will agree. The FMV assumes prevailing economic and market conditions and is calculated based on multiple factors, including practice characteristics such as location, area demographics, referral base, and cost of operations or overhead; cost of physical site and business and dental equipment; cost of software and related licenses (including transfer of existing licenses); costs related to maintenance and

Table 1
Advisory team professionals and their functions

Professionals	Function
Financial consultant/accounting firm	Practice valuation
	Tax implications advise
	Preparing cash flow and break-even projections
	Payroll setup and management
	Bookkeeping
	Filing of taxes
Attorney/legal services	Negotiating purchase contracts
	Reviewing lease or rental agreements
	Licensure and other compliance
	Liability matters
	Claims management
	Reviewing and negotiating associateship contracts
Management consultants	Transition management
	Coordinating advisors
	Staff communications
	Staffing, scheduling, policy development
	Writing manuals/policies
	Risk management
	Marketing and promotional activities
	Daily operational activities
Insurance specialists	Assisting in buying/selling of insurance
	Medical malpractice and liability insurance
	Billing errors and omissions insurance
	Employment practice liability
	Worker's compensation
	Disability insurance
	Health insurance for self and employees
	Other insurance matters (business policy, life insurance, long-term care)
Banker	Mortgage processing
	Loan and credit facilitation (provide accessible funds for the business venture)
Realtor	Finding suitable office and housing
Financial planner	Helping with savings and investments
	Preparing retirement proposals
	Protecting against business loss
	Developing succession strategies
Others	Architect or interior designer
	Contractor to remodel or construct office

lease contracts (including transfer or renegotiation of existing contracts); profitability; and market considerations. It also considers other reasonable assumptions of practice performance based on the current dentist's patient records, longevity of practice, and *goodwill*, which may be broadly defined as professional reputation, contacts, and relationships. Thus, valuation is a process through which a purchase price is allocated to various tangible and intangible assets, such as equipment, supplies, leasehold improvements, noncompete covenant, patient records, and goodwill.

In addition to the FMV of the practice, other considerations may impact a decision to purchase.

Cash and accounts receivable

Case and accounts receivable are distinct from FMV and are properties of the seller that can be negotiated for separately. *Accounts receivable* refers to outstanding collections owed to the buyer at the time of purchase and is typically discounted based on industry standards on aging of past-due accounts and estimation of reasonably collectible value.

Outstanding liabilities

Outstanding liabilities include accounts and taxes payable at the time of purchase. It is important to confirm that the current owner will settle all liabilities before the transfer. If not, these liabilities must be deducted from purchase price.

Automobiles or other vehicles

Automobiles or other vehicles belonging to the owner, if available for purchase, are not typically included in FMV assessments and must be negotiated independently.

Personal effects

Certain personal effects, such as artwork, decorative items, and music CDs, may be additional assets that will not be included in FMV assessments and require independent decisions to purchase in whole or part.

A valuation consultant or accounting firm can help prepare a valuation report. The report is typically commissioned by the practice owner's representative or appraiser and is useful to sellers and buyers. It helps the seller establish an asking price for the practice, and helps the buyer establish a bidding price for the practice and provides valid documentation in securing financing for the purchase. Box 1 lists the components and benefits of establishing an FMV.

Buyers must review the fair market assessment report before deciding to purchase. Obtaining an independent buyer's evaluation may also be helpful in decision making [1].

Purchasing an established practice: step-by-step guide

Purchase of an established practice involves multiple considerations. A buyer's due diligence should include market and demographics research (eg, dentist-to-population ratios, local economy, area hospitals and surgical facilities), consideration of FMV, assessment of opportunities for

Box 1. Components and benefits of establishing fair market value of a dental practice

Components of valuation

Fair market value

- Referral history and base
- Procedure fees
- Reasonable estimation of earnings
- Lease/purchase cost for physical site
- Cost of tangible and intangible assets
- Overhead/operating costs
- Wages, taxes, benefits
- Insurance costs
- Equipment lease/rentals/current costs
- Cost of maintenance and license agreements
- Depreciation and amortization
- Continuing education

Other factors

- Working capital
- Acquisition cost
- Debt servicing

Benefits to the seller

- Helps establish selling price
- May be used as marketing tool when selling the practice
- Helps assure financial solvency of the practice

Benefits to the buyer

- Provides the basis for buy/no-buy decision
- Establishes realistic framework to ascertain whether he/she can cover expenses, have a reasonable income and/or profit, and be able to repay loans in a reasonable period of time
- Provides documentation for loan applications and improves chances of acquiring financing for the purchase

professional development, and personal considerations. The following items may help provide a framework on which modifications can be imposed to meet individual situations and preferences [1–3].

Selecting a community/geographic area

Selecting a community or geographic area is largely based on personal and family considerations. However, factors such as availability of staffing and operating privileges, and continuing education opportunities will be important to assure that one can keep current with developments in the field and develop a professional network.

Arranging advisory team

Once the geographic location is known, the next step is to begin establishing an advisory team. A practice purchase and management consultant and realtor are some of the first professionals that may be useful in this regard. Others may be added as appropriate as the evaluation and purchase process progresses. The ADA provides many useful directories that can be a good resource for identifying qualified professionals.

Finding an available practice

As an early step, practices for sale in the preferred community should be investigated. This search is important, because it may help determine whether purchasing an existing practice is a viable option. Classified advertisements in professional journals, hospital bulletin boards, Web searches, and word-of-mouth are all viable sources for this information. A local real estate agent may also be useful (see Table 1).

Initiating discovery and discussion

Once a practice has been identified, a confidentiality agreement must be signed and an initial on-site interview arranged with the seller and seller's agent. This encounter will provide an opportunity to meet and establish a rapport with the seller. An initial site inspection can also occur at this time. Furthermore, mutual goals, objectives, and timeframes can be discussed and any questions about the practice and sale terms, financing, and transitioning process can be clarified. The buyer should come prepared with potential questions and, if interested in pursuing further, obtain a copy of the confidential valuation report from the seller or seller's agent [1].

Evaluating and making an offer

The advisors should then review and appraise the valuation report, and a consultant may perform an independent valuation if the preliminary review seems promising. The valuation consultants should be able to prepare a cash flow analysis, conduct a site visit, and determine a fair price for purchase of practice (note that this may differ from FMV) (see Table 1). The consultant will also be able to clarify any doubts or questions with the seller. Once the buyer is satisfied, a formal purchase offer should be made through the legal representative or consultant.

Proceeding with the sale–purchase in good faith

Once a purchase offer is signed by both parties, it is considered fully executed and the buyer provides a down payment or deposits funds into escrow. This activity conveys a good faith intention to purchase (contingent on acquisition of appropriate licensing, lease agreements, financing) and takes the practice off the market. The seller's attorney generally drafts a comprehensive Agreement of Sale.

At this point, the buyer should review the agreement with the attorney (see Table 1), who may further discuss and negotiate alterations to the agreement with the seller's attorney until both parties are satisfied. Once the agreement is signed by both parties, preparation for closing the deal can begin.

Preparing for purchase closure

Obtaining adequate financing and insurance coverage and achieving regulatory compliance are crucial next steps in preparing to close the deal and transition to the new practice. Financing can be a complicated process; preparation of support documents can be critical and save time and money. Developing a finance packet and approaching several banks/lending institutions for a loan may be a good idea. Alternatively, the buyer may approach the seller if the option of financing the deal was indicated.

A finance packet typically includes a business plan; the buyer's *curriculum vitae*, credit rating, tax returns, and personal budgets; the facility lease copy, a copy of the signed agreement of sale, and other specific documents requested by the target bank or institution. An accountant or practice management professional can help in this process (see Table 1).

This process will be time-consuming; buyers should prepare for this interim period by having or obtaining working capital and a line of credit for payment of immediate bills (eg, rent, utilities, wages, telephone) and personal maintenance during the set-up phase and before opening the practice. Generally, the working capital should be sufficient to cover at least 2 to 3 months of expenses.

Once a loan application is provisionally approved, other items such as insurance and licenses must be established. This phase is a good time to complete applications for Medicare participation, confirm that all license requirements are met, and transfer the DEA number. Next, buyers may transfer or apply for professional liability or malpractice insurance, including tail coverage. Finally, buyers should ensure other necessary insurance plans are in place, such as insurance for office liability; worker's compensation and unemployment; health care; automobile; and loan reduction In other words, this phase of preparation assures that the buyer has completed the needed financial, legal, and compliance documentation.

Preparing to launch practice

Next, steps should be initiated to help launch the new practice. The practice cannot exist in isolation; buyers must establish relationships with local medical institutions and obtain staff privileges in local hospitals/clinics. If the practice is being purchased from a well-established dentist, he may help facilitate this process.

It may be a good idea and a professional courtesy to compose and distribute introductory letters to other professionals in the area. This gesture will serve as the new practice's presentation to the professional community.

Buyers should explore the community and review all marketing opportunities that may be useful in targeting future patients (eg, local newspapers, specialty advertising periodicals, yellow pages, online directories, local community Web sites). Management consultants should be helpful in directing and reviewing options (see Table 1). They will also be helpful in developing marketing material, such as brochures, advertisements, fliers, and announcements targeted to patients and other relevant individuals/companies about the upcoming change or succession from the previous dentist, and highlighting areas of the new practice.

Reviewing and updating any existing directory listings and advertisements related to the current practice may also be useful. New stationery, signage, records, forms, and supplies must also be obtained, and the fee structure reviewed and updated as needed.

A key part of any dental practice is the staff. Part of any successful conversion will involve a transition of existing staff from the previous practice. Buyers should review policy and personnel manuals with a management consultant to ensure familiarity; this also provides an opportunity for any necessary aspects to be updated or changed.

Buyers should work with the seller to discuss staff and rehire or transition individuals who may continue in the new practice. Retaining old staff can have many advantages: they know the old patients, are familiar with the community, are probably already trained and experienced, and are generally motivated to retain their employment.

However, some disadvantages must be recognized, including reluctance to change and loyalty, policies, or practices. Staff transition should therefore be handled sensitively, and it will be important to work with each member individually to convey the new philosophies, goals, and practice. The staff will require reassurance regarding employment, security, and other uncertainties they may associate with the transition. Enlisting help from the seller and management professionals will help ease the transition for everyone.

Closing the deal and transitioning to the new practice

Once funding is finalized and all other preparations are complete, the purchase can be closed with final sign-off on the sale contract and transfer of assets to the new owner. Legal and financial advisors review all documents before they are signed. The independent practice is now ready to be started. Although challenges may be anticipated, ethical practice will ensure personal and professional satisfaction. Periodically, goals should be monitored, staff reviews conducted, and the practice evaluated for quality assurance. The ADA is a good resource for updating skills and keeping current with practice tools and legal and ethical issues.

Opting for an associateship

Based on personal and personality considerations, an associateship (ie, practicing in association with other dentists in a group setting) may be a better option for some. Associateship can occur in different forms: as an employee or independent contractor, or as a colleague who has space-, expense-, and time-sharing options. These forms do not always have an option for equity ownership.

The most conventional form of associateship is one leading to equity ownership in the practice (buy-in option). This option can be more comfortable for individuals who wish to acclimatize to a practice or practice area before making a purchase investment.

This type of ownership can generally be divided into three phases: (1) a break-in/trial phase; (2) a buy-in phase; and (3) a buy-out phase. The duration of each phase and the terms of the buy-in (partnership) and buy-out phases (ownership) are determined and agreed on at the start of the associateship. Practice valuation and establishment of future purchase price also occur at this time. The overall steps (Fig. 1) involved in an associateship with a buy-in option generally include the many steps discussed earlier for an outright purchase and are briefly summarized in this section, highlighting key elements of this option [1,2].

Locating an appropriate practice

As with an outright purchase, personal and professional factors determine the preferred practice location.

Initial interview

During the initial review with the senior dentist or partner, one should be prepared to outline the compensation requirements, such as reasonable income compensation, annual incentives, initial employment term, and benefits, including insurances, vacations, continuing education, and auto allowances. The initial interview is an opportunity to establish mutual compatibility and obtain and provide references. This interview typically lasts a few hours and may occur on- or off-site.

Second interview

If both parties wish to proceed beyond the first interview, the second interview should be planned to occur on-site so that the potential associate has an opportunity to review the location and general geographic area, review the facility, and meet the staff and other associates. Assignments of patients, types of cases that might be seen, and potential for participation in managing the practice can be discussed. Profit-sharing opportunities, retirement benefits, and buy-in and buy-out options are also appropriate to discuss at this phase.

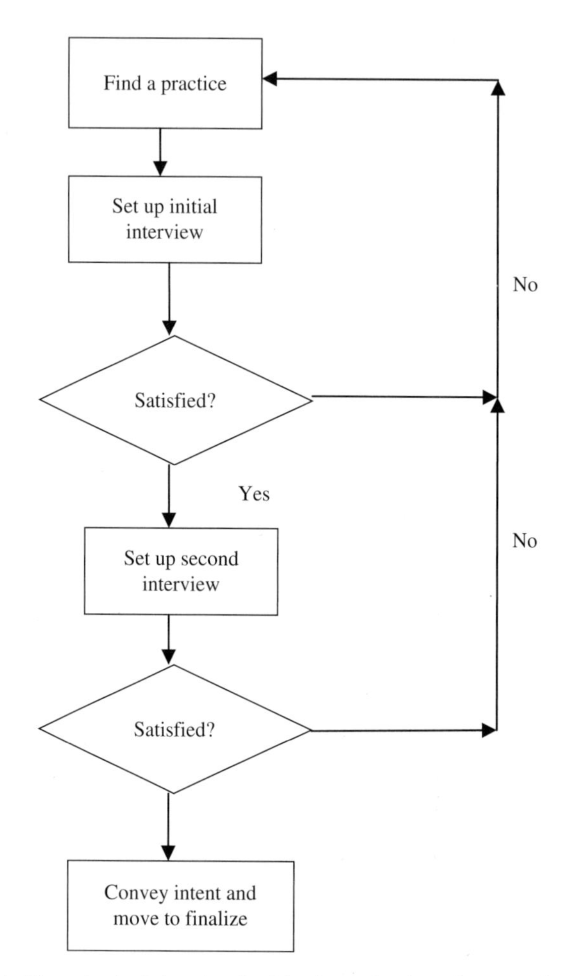

Fig. 1. Flow-chart of steps involved in the evaluation of an associateship.

Conveying intent and finalizing

If satisfied, potential associates should convey their intent to join the practice. This stage should prompt an official Letter of Intent from the senior dentist based on the terms discussed during the interviews. In some cases, a third meeting may be organized and expanded to included spouses and other family members; this is a good opportunity for all individuals to familiarize themselves with the upcoming changes and prepare for move.

Both parties must sign off on the associateship contract before it can be final. A legal advisor should be retained who can review all documents and negotiate any changes. After sign-off by both parties, the new member will be ready to start the first phase of the associateship. The new associate should expect to periodically review the status of the associateship and to proceed to the buy-in and buy-out phases according to the contract.

Summary

Evaluating a dental practice for outright purchase or associateship is exciting for a dentist. It can be a long and complicated process but, with appropriate preparation and help of qualified advisors, can be satisfying and lead to a successful and fulfilling career and life. Obtaining the help of appropriate and trustworthy advisors is key to successful navigation of the evaluation, buying, and contracting processes.

Also important is an ability to effectively communicate with and coordinate all advisors and activities. Being prepared and open and considerate of the other party's viewpoint, and acting ethically and professionally are key to success. Underestimating the time and effort required to find the right site or practice, and to complete negotiations and transition to the new practice is a common pitfall and source of discouragement; this can be avoided by being aware of the overall process and having realistic expectations.

Other pitfalls to avoid include insufficient planning and inadequate preparation or insensitivity to the transitioning process. It is hoped that the steps outlined in this paper will help facilitate passage across this important milestone and help assure success and fulfillment.

References

[1] American Dental Association. Valuing a practice: a guide for dentists.

[2] Pollack SL. Entering an ethical and successful oral and maxillofacial surgical practice. Oral Maxillofac Surg Clin North Am 1999;11(3):377–90.

[3] Snyder T. How to buy a dental practice. Available at: http://www.dentalcompare.com/featuredarticle.asp?articleid=273. Accessed February 6, 2008.

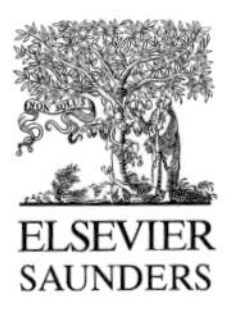

Dent Clin N Am 52 (2008) 495–505

THE DENTAL CLINICS OF NORTH AMERICA

Management and Marketing for the General Practice Dental Office

Earl Clarkson, DDS*,
Sanjeev Bhatia, DDS, FDS RCS(Eng), MDS

Department of Oral and Maxillofacial Surgery, The Brooklyn Hospital Center, 121 Dekalb Avenue, Brooklyn, NY 11201, USA

The public has a general awareness that the aim of dental practitioners is to help patients maintain dental and oral health throughout life. In a Harris Poll, in May 2006, of United States adults regarding whom they trust most, dentists ranked near the top of the list among providers in all health care and non–health care related fields [1]. The degree of trust that patients have for dentists reflects the success of the patient-centered dental practice model; patients are included in the decision-making process regarding their own oral health. Marketing is the first step in patient education. As evidenced by the increasing number of new treatment modalities, including new technologies for minimally invasive and cosmetic dentistry, dentistry is a dynamic field in health care. Marketing the new techniques available in dentistry gives dental patients a greater range of choice and control over the care they receive. Furthermore, rather than focusing solely on one area of dental disease that may be the presenting the chief complaint, patients must come to see that optimal dental health is a year-round endeavor influencing systemic health. The Surgeon General's Report on oral health in the United States brought to the forefront data linking oral health and overall systemic health and correlating periodontal disease with low and pre-term birth weight [2]. The message of the Surgeon General from 2000 is just as true today. Reinforcing the message of the oral health and systemic link and the need for preventative and restorative care is part of the goal of proper marketing.

A good marketing message for a practice is targeted to a specific group of patients. Marketing should demonstrate the capacity of a practice to satisfy patients' specific needs. Dental practices that offer specific services in the

* Corresponding author.
E-mail address: eicddsoms@yahoo.com (E. Clarkson).

doi:10.1016/j.cden.2008.03.003

areas of pediatric care, periodontal procedures, oral surgery, or orthodontics should highlight these areas as strengths of a practice through marketing. Many practices today emphasize offering cosmetic procedures, such as veneers and bleaching, because these often are key areas of interest among new patients as they have a dramatic effect on appearance and the psychologic outlook of patients. Thus, each dental practice has an identity determined by the scope and strengths of a practitioner. Dentists continue to expand the scope of practice through continuing education throughout their careers, and marketing should reflect the new offerings of a dental practice. The best marketing of a dental practice highlights the unique characteristics of the practice. The level of experience of dentists in a practice, including any additional training attained, should be advertised. The hours of a practice, including any weekend hours, should be listed as patients are drawn to the convenience of additional hours of operation. Marketing a practice's identity—the skill of the practitioner and services offered—allows patients to understand how a practice fits their specific needs.

Managing a dental practice requires an understanding of marketing the services provided, which leads to economic sustainability for the dental practice. To have a more quantitative approach to the running of a dental practice, key performance indicators (KPIs) may be used by a dental practice to track the success of a marketing message. KPIs have long been used by businesses in non–health care sectors to gauge the financial status of a business [3]. General dental practice owners must understand whether or not the number of patients is increasing or decreasing and whether or not patients treated are having greater or fewer numbers of services provided. The financial success of a dental practice also depends on the remuneration provided by patients through dental insurance or fee for services delivered. Knowledge of KPIs, the vital signs of a dental practice, gives a practice owner a sense of the current financial health of the practice. In addition to the current state of a practice, the effect of all decisions made from hiring new employees to purchasing new equipment and treatment space may be gauged preliminarily through KPIs [4].

The mission statement and management plan

Strategic planning is an important part of guiding the direction of a dental practice. The formal plan for a practice is based on a global mission statement. The long-term practice goals should be written to include a practice's philosophy. The long-term goals also should include a vision of how a practice will be run when it is passed on to a future dentist or sold. The equity built into a practice is part of a successful long-term goal. In formulating a mission statement, a dentist should list general goals of the practice initially, followed by specific objectives in the immediate term. Statement of objectives should be in a clear and concise fashion, firmly establishing the goal to be accomplished. Foremost, objectives must be realistic and achievable. The objective must be achievable within a prescribed time frame. Next, individual planned actions should be listed, such as increased marketing of certain areas of the practice. Strategic planning is an ongoing part of building a successful practice. Each quarter, the plan should be revised based on the degree of success of practice decisions made. A mission statement and the work ethic it embodies translate into a comfortable, positive clinic environment for patients. Such an environment leads to the most cost-effective marketing: word-of-mouth referrals. Word-of-mouth referrals are an invaluable part of any dental practice marketing plan.

A practice vision process (outlined previously) initially requires establishing a general vision, mission, and values of a practice. Such a vision might be to provide comprehensive care with emphasis on patient satisfaction with the esthetics of the smile while ensuring that the oral health of patients is maintained. The next step in the mission statement is to define key strategic goals. The methods for achieving the strategic goals are discussed next in the statement. Each quarter, the methods should be re-evaluated to determine if they have been successful.

The objectives, or KPIs, of the management plan should be measurable. For example, a practicing dentist may aim to increase the number of patients returning for periodontal maintenance therapy as scheduled. At least one indicator should be used that is measurable to ascertain the accomplishment of the objective [5]. In this case, the number of patients returning is a readily measurable quantity. The number of active patients seen in a dental practice is another KPI. Although many investments, such as investment in equipment, depreciate over time, increasing numbers of patients visiting a practice allows a practice to appreciate in value [6]. Not only do additional patients bring added value to a practice, they help to spread the word about the quality of the work performed at a practice through word-of-mouth referrals. Auditing the relationships a practitioner has with influential members of the community gives a sense of how a practice is faring in the intangible but important area of practice reputation.

Marketing objectives

Marketing objectives may span a range of purposes and should challenge dentists and staffs daily to work toward specific goals. The challenge of the stated objectives leads to a greater commitment to a practice. As shown repeatedly in studies, workers who are given specific goals work harder and have a greater sense of satisfaction in their daily work [7]. Objectives build practice unity by helping to bring all members of a practice staff together in seeking to achieve a specific goal. The challenges must be realistic but attainable. Acknowledging objectives as they are obtained gives the members of a practice a sense of accomplishment. Besides leading to a greater sense of fulfillment by staff, the focus on specific objectives leads to greater efficiency. When all members are working toward concrete goals, efforts are concentrated and coordinated so that staff are not working against each other. Continued productivity is encouraged when members who are particularly successful at attaining practice goals are rewarded and incentives are given for goals that are achieved.

Marketing audits

The first step in a marketing planning process is conducting an initial marketing audit. Don Sheelen, Chief Executive Officer of the 100 year-old Regina Vacuum Cleaner Company, states, "a complete marketing audit is an absolutely essential step; without it, your chances of success are cut in half" [8]. The current methods of marketing should be compared with marketing methods known to be successful. An initial assessment should bring attention to areas that are deficient. Special attention should be given to areas considered critically deficient that have hampered the growth of a practice. Such areas might include poor communication with patients or staff. There should be common elements of courtesy extended to each patient, and all staff members should practice making patients feel comfortable from initial encounters to follow-up after discharge [9]. Ultimately, the best measure of marketing success is the level of patient satisfaction. Simple daily habits, such as asking how patients are feeling and thanking patients for coming in, may be the best way to retain patients and improve the patient experience.

An initial marketing audit captures the initial picture of a practice's state. In a tightly knit organization, like a dental office, there are a few elements that have greatest impact on a marketing plan. Some of the key areas for the initial audit are establishing characteristics of the patient base and how patients are referred to a practice. Unique characteristics of the patients served and specific needs and services desired by these patients also are important. The expectations of patients are particularly important. The perceptions of patients should be described, including their attitudes toward the provided services, including cosmetic and other restorative services. Listed, in order, an initial audit should establish

- The patients served
- Key characteristics of these patients
- Characteristics that differentiate these patients from other patients
- Patients' needs and wants
- Patients' expectations
- Special requirements and perceptions
- Feedback on dental services and care environment
- Attitudes toward oral health
- Oral health, cosmetic, and dental needs

Success of a dental practice depends on patients feeling satisfied with the treatment options offered and the quality with which those services are delivered. The patient experience extends beyond the dental chair, and the practice staff must be encouraged to foster a positive atmosphere of care for patients in all areas of a clinic. Staff members should be made to feel they are stakeholders in the success of the practice and that their conduct influences the manner in which patients view the practice [9].

Marketing objectives

James Quinn, in *Strategies for Change: Logical Incrementalism*, defines objectives as a statement of "what is to be achieved and when results are to be accomplished but not *how* the results are to be achieved" [10]. A marketing planning process begins with stating objectives of a practice. Marketing objectives state just where a dental office intends to be at a specific time in the future. Sheelen writes that objectives must be "measurable and office members must be held accountable to their specific goals" [9]. To be effective, objectives should be capable of measurement: quantifiable. The measurement may be in terms of numbers of patients, patient compliance and satisfaction, or financial indicators. An example of a measurable marketing objective is capturing 10% of the market for dental whitening services during 1 year. The bleaching techniques should be outlined in the objective and the expected results in terms of numbers of patients seeking the services should be listed. In addition, the income generated should be described. Marketing objectives include a dental practice's financial objectives. Once quantified, the goal may be monitored unequivocally and corrections may be made as progress toward the objective is made. The objectives list which products or services are available from a practice and what is the desired penetration of the market for these services.

External and internal marketing

Once strategy and objectives are laid out, the process of implementation begins through marketing. Effective marketing of a dental practice is through a combination of advertising methods aimed at spreading the word about a practice within the community. Taken together, multimedia Web pages, magazines, and direct mail all may contribute to advertising but usually are not as effective individually as they are when used together. Targeting advertising is the most effective at attracting patients who have preidentified needs or desired procedures to a practice. Specific advertising methods and their advantages and disadvantages are outlined.

Informative and promotional pamphlets

A newsletter or promotional pamphlet may help a practice spread the word about services offered. A pamphlet describing the services offered may be read by patients in a waiting room. Patients waiting to be treated thus may be informed about additional services offered by a practice. Patients who are waiting are a receptive audience for such informative material. Current information regarding office hours, new staff, and equipment purchased may be communicated to patients through pamphlets in the waiting room or sent by mail. The brochures may contain patient testimonials and pictures of successful cases, and citations of available research help to convince patients of the safety and efficacy of certain procedures. Patients should be encouraged to take brochures that have pictures of office staff and general information regarding directions to the office, telephone numbers, and the range of services offered with them to share with other potential patients. The disadvantage of published materials, such as pamphlets and brochures, is that they often are prohibitively expensive to produce.

Outreach

Some of the best advertising is through involvement of a dentist and staff with local and national organizations. Involvement in the community is a valuable form of networking. Educational seminars and lectures for community groups are another opportunity to advertise the work of a practice. Lectures given at hospitals, religious institutions, and clubs are a direct method of communicating with potential patients. Maintaining a list of attendees for an RSVP list allows follow-up with written promotional materials. There are a multitude of outreach activities that increase the visibility of a practice in the community. Donating time to help meet a need in the community also may lead to positive word of mouth referrals. Having a practice associated with such worthy causes establishes a link between the practice and positive efforts by the community.

Advertising in the telephone book

The best advertising in the Yellow Pages is through a simple but professionally designed advertisement. An advertisement should state clearly all information necessary to finding a practice. An advertisement should be attractive to potential patients and help patients find the office and know its hours of operation. All services of specific interest to the patients in the community should be displayed clearly in an advertisement. Hours of practice and forms of payment accepted by a practice are useful for patients in an advertisement.

Advertising in newspapers and magazines

A practice gains valuable exposure through advertisements placed in local newspapers and magazines. Targeting advertising to fit with the typical audience for the publication ensures a receptive audience. A magazine about wedding planning is an excellent place to discuss cosmetic and esthetic dentistry, such as veneers and tooth whitening. Such advertisements often are expensive, however, and may be an addition to rather than a staple of regular advertising.

The Internet

The telephone book, a good source of self-referrals, no longer is the leading source of referrals for most dental practices. For most patients in the United States, the Internet is one of the first sources checked for information about local dentists. Patients use the Internet to retrieve information about practitioners. Patients during these times usually are investigating elective procedures, so establishing a presence on the Web not only attracts these patients during times when only an elective desire for dental services exists but also establishes a connection with patients for times of immediate need for dental care [11,12]. Well-designed Web sites may help dental practitioners accomplish many of the things essential to building a practice. Web sites may streamline administrative tasks, allowing for better patient follow-up and higher patient satisfaction. Much that is involved with patient registration and education may be offered through the Internet. A receptionist may direct patients to a practice's Web site before their initial visit.

Multimedia resources

Through Macromedia Flash and other computer programs, general dentists may create a variety of effective marketing presentations. These multimedia advertisements may be sent through e-mail or be displayed to patients during treatment planning sessions. Beyond the basic information about location of a practice and hours of operation, a presentation my inform patients about the availability of emergency care, scheduling procedures, and treatment planning.

Internal marketing

Internal marketing begins in the office. The atmosphere a dental practitioner creates within an office influences patients' perceptions of a practice. A practitioner and all auxiliary staff must maintain a professional and caring atmosphere in a practice. A memorable, distinctive logo that reflects the ideals of a practice is a symbol that patients find easy to remember when thinking about the practice. A logo may be used on stationery, prescription forms, invitations, uniforms, and all other forms of communication with the public. The cleanliness of a clinic and sterility of instruments is paramount to the perception of a clinic as well run. Informing patients about a practice's careful adherence to sterility guidelines is important to maintaining trust with patients. Insulate patients from the sounds of treatment rooms and staff conversations. Keep patients' information confidential, including keeping conversations private. Another area in which practitioners may gain trust with patients is through financial assistance with payment options and divided payment plans. Patient satisfaction and follow-through on treatment recommendations improves if patients have a choice of payment options. A staff member well versed in dental insurance matters may help patients obtain coverage. Treatment guarantees and free consultations can smooth the way for reluctant patients. Telephone, front-desk, and postoperative etiquette determine patients' view of a practice's responsiveness. Few things put patients off as much as being kept on hold; incorporate promotional information into messages when a short wait is necessary. Having a receptionist call before an appointment and with a follow-up makes a favorable impression. Create a log to keep tract of patients' calls and what the calls are about. Try to make sure potential patients are not ignored. If necessary, send additional information to patients.

Employee relations

Choosing the correct employees is essential to the success of a dental practice. Staff must have the same vision as the practitioner and be capable of performing the necessary steps to attain it. They should be energetic and friendly, enjoy their careers, and be community conscious. It is important to adopt corporate management strategies in dealing with hiring and termination of staff. Poor hiring and termination practices can lead to high employee turnover on doctor stress. Consider employee manuals that adhere to state, local, and federal principles. Poor human resource skills may lead to lawsuits as a result of wrongful discharge, sexual harassment, or discrimination. Sexual harassment suits can ruin the reputation of the doctor, destroy office morale, and cost millions of dollars. They are not covered by malpractice or umbrella insurance. Do not hire family members, spouses, or friends as employees. They can be problematic in the future, difficult to terminate, and create employee problems. Consultation and summer help are exceptions. Doctor-employee relationships should remain just that. Inappropriate contacts, racial jokes, or commenting on attire or physical traits can lead to lawsuits. Do not manipulate monetary funds; in other words, do not try to avoid taxes. There should be some distance between a doctor's personal or family life and what the staff knows.

Specialty outlook

General dentists are responsible for the bulk of referrals to specialty practices even in today's wired world. Much of the focus for internal marketing for specialists should be to maintaining and nurturing a healthy relationship with a general practitioner (GP). Approximately 60% to 95% of referrals are made by general dentists. Referrals from patients, dental specialists, medical practitioners, friends, allied health providers, health maintenance organizations, and staff contribute the remainder of patients to a specialist's office. The changing dynamics of dental marketing has created a new competitive market for dentistry. In this new age of competition, specialists need to understand this business end of their practice.

Marketing concepts

One of the critical elements in this business is the understanding and adoption of marketing concepts. Marketing concepts are straightforward; that is, to market a practice effectively, patients' needs and dentists' needs must be identified and understood and solutions developed that satisfy both. In a specialty practice, the perspective has to have the orientation that whatever is done, is done with patients in mind. This belief, that they are the center of marketing strategy, should be vibrant in every aspect of the business.

Working with a marketing consultant can be helpful when a practice has an objective of substantial growth or protecting business investment against potential attrition or loss of patients to more competitive marketing by other practices. A good marketing company is important because it can look at a practice in terms of strategic planning. Once specialists have their clinical skills in place and a practice is financially stable, it could be considered a smart move to recruit a consultant for the marketing aspects of practice building.

Referral levels are increased because a practice takes time to market effectively. It also is significant that a marketing program functions at several levels. Just look at how often a receptionist speaks to another receptionist at the referring office. If practitioners realize the incredible capability of staff and invest in their training, they can play a major role in marketing and communication process. Remember, GP staffs play an influential role in deciding where patients may be referred. It has been seen that four out of five GP patients ask a clinical question of a staff person. Certainly, many were, "Which specialist is the best?"

Set up a calendar for the year to plan out all marketing programs. Analyze each program to be sure objectives specified in the marketing messages can be met; by establishing a plan, each phase of a marketing program can be prepared for. Coordinating with staff and gaining momentum for the program help increase the chances of the program's implementation. A fixed amount of finances should be set aside to be used for marketing, because having a fixed dollar amount creates a feeling of responsibility to spend that money. A staff member should be identified who is responsible for performing the marketing program. Staff should be engaged in staff marketing.

Establish a budget for the receptionist to take other receptionists to lunch or send fruit baskets or flowers to GP staffs in appreciation. The ability to involve staff and assign specific individuals responsibilities in planning a marketing program is a powerful team-building tool and enhances the marketing effort.

The goal of all marketing is to have an effect. The dynamics of specialty practice marketing continue to evolve. As diagnostics and treatment modalities become more integrated between a GP and a specialty practice, future marketing focuses more heavily of the cohesive team-oriented relationship. There are many examples where orthodontics, oral and maxillofacial surgery (OMFS), implant surgery, and medical specialties must be coordinated. Orthognathic surgery requires OMFS, GP, and orthodontist coordination. Implants require the OMFS, GP, and laboratory personnel in most cases. There are cases where an OMFS sends a patient back to a GP for final esthetic enhancement or occlusal therapy. To enhance long-term relationships, a specialist should be as specific about the needs of each office as possible. Specialists and GPs should try to know each other by knowing more about each other's interests. This promotes welcome conversation on the telephone or in person. People love to refer to their friends, and friends have an interest in one another.

One excellent strategy for following-up on the success of a marketing program to referring offices is to continuously assess the generalized impact. The OMFS should make it a point to ask referring dentists in various settings if the OMFS practice is providing service commensurate with the needs and desires of the GP. It is worthwhile to encourage staff to occasionally ask the staff of the GP the same types of questions. By discovering a problem early via a marketing follow-up process, there is an excellent chance to solve the problem before a general dentist begins to refer elsewhere. Remember to target marketing for the accomplishment of specific goals. Each month or year, a different set of marketing strategies can be used with the underlying principle that all contacts with GPs are of a highly positive nature. Do not make the mistake of waiting until a practice has slowed down to begin marketing. As competition increases for specialty services, it is important to keep a specialist's message clearly at the top of a GP's mind.

One area that has increased productivity for many specialist practices is dental implants, especially for oral surgery. Some OMFS practices have set a goal to increase referrals for implants. One of the strategies they use is study clubs. A specialist can start or sponsor evening courses ranging from implant placement to home care hygiene for implant patients. There are many people who enjoy speaking at a study club. The key to a successful study club is finding someone who can take responsibility for organizing and perpetuating a group. Furthermore, staff can be involved in helping to get a study club to work. They would enjoy interaction with a GP and the excitement of implant emphasis. The GP's staff can be invited to meetings they might enjoy. GPs can be invited to seminars sponsored by specialists with help of an implant company representative to expose referring dentists to surgical and restorative techniques. These could be cosponsored with a dental laboratory. Special forms for implant referrals forms can be created and distributed to every potential dentist, making referral easy and convenient. Various strategies should be defined and implemented to reach a patient population and to position a practice in the competitive market.

Successful management and marketing of a dental practice requires a systematic process of setting objectives, auditing KPIs, and drawing new patients through advertising. The range of treatment choices offered by dentists is growing and patients are seeking an increasing number of elective procedures. Keeping patients healthy and happy is the best method to promote a successful general dental practice.

References

[1] The Harris Poll. Doctors, dentists and nurses most trusted professionals to give advice: poll of adults in the United States. Available at: http://info@harrisinteractive.com.
[2] U.S. Department of Health and Human Services. Oral health in America: a report of the Surgeon General. Rockville (MD): National Institute of Dental and Craniofacial Research; 2000.
[3] Levin RL. The business of dentistry: a better practice. J Am Dent Assoc 2003;134(5):644–5.
[4] Levin RL. The business of dentistry, a better practice. J Am Dent Assoc 2003;134(5):645.
[5] Wilson A. The marketing of professional services. New York: Mc-Graw Hill; 1972.
[6] McGuigan PJ, Eisner AB. Marketing the dental practice: eight steps toward success. J Am Dent Assoc 2006;137:1426–33.
[7] McGuigan, Levin RL, et al. Developing a data base to increase referrals. PM Notes—August 91 Digest.
[8] Wells JT. Timing is of the essence. Online Journal of Accountancy. Available at: http://www.aicpa.org/pubs/jofa/joahome.htm. Accessed February 13, 2008.
[9] Wells, May 2001.
[10] Quinn JB. 1980 strategies for change: logical incrementalism. In: Irwin R, Reich RB, editors. The next American frontier. New York: Times Books; 1983.
[11] Paroha K. Marketing for the dental professional. The Vital Resource; 1991.
[12] Niamtu J. Marketing the oral and maxillofacial surgery practice,"anesthesia/dentoalveolar surgery/office management". In: Fonsera RJ, editor. Form of practice in dentistry, ADA. W.B. Saunders Company; 1990.

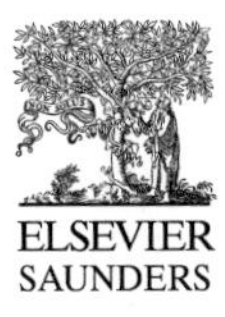

ELSEVIER
SAUNDERS

Dent Clin N Am 52 (2008) 507–527

THE DENTAL
CLINICS
OF NORTH AMERICA

Insurance Billing and Coding

Rebecca H. Napier[a], Lori S. Bruelheide[b], Eric T.K. Demann, DMD[c,*], Richard H. Haug, DDS[d]

[a]*Department of Surgery, University of Kentucky, College of Dentistry, D-508, 800 Rose Street, Lexington, KY 40536–0297, USA*
[b]*University of Kentucky, College of Dentistry, Kentucky Clinic Dentistry, M-128, 800 Rose Street, Lexington, KY 40536, USA*
[c]*University of Kentucky, College of Dentistry, Kentucky Clinic Dentistry, A-219, Lexington, KY 40536–0284, USA*
[d]*University of Kentucky, College of Dentistry, D-136, 800 Rose Street; Room, Lexington, KY 40536–0297, USA*

Codes—what are they? And why do we use them?

International Classification of Diseases, Ninth Revision, Clinical Modification (ICD.9.CM), current procedural terminology (CPT), and common dental terminology (CDT) codes are merely a series of numbers (numeric) or letters and numbers (alpha-numeric) that are used to identify a condition, malady, disease process, etiology, procedure, or management modality. Although "one picture is worth a thousand words," the use of one code can save the use of dozens of words. Codes are more concise than long descriptions; provide a more uniform means of communication; and bridge the gap between different languages, geographic connotations, and differences in profession, specialty, or subspecialty. They can be used to save time and space while charting or to collect demographic and frequency data for research; however, codes are a must for billing.

Billing

The advancement of medical technology throughout the twentieth century dictated a revolution of medical science. Innovation in medicine increased not only consumption of health care services but the cost of medical care, and subsequently created an increased financial responsibility for the

* Corresponding author.
E-mail address: edemann@yahoo.com (E.T.K. Demann).

doi:10.1016/j.cden.2008.02.008

patient, or end-consumer. This fiscal amplification produced public demand for privately held health insurance to balance and mitigate the risk for significant health care expenditure. As third-party payers began to shoulder the financial responsibility of medical care, the need was identified to interpret, classify, and establish work and reimbursement values for medical procedures submitted by myriad health care practitioners from diverse specialties, geographic areas, and training backgrounds. Standardized billing practices, in the form of uniform coding–consistent forms and documents, provide a mechanism for health care practitioners to submit succinct yet precise accounts of services rendered to third-party payers. Consistency of coding and formatting for claims permits the immediate and accurate interpretation of those services by the payer, overcoming common communication barriers. More than 500 million claims are filed to third-party health plans each month in the United States [1], a volume mandating the elimination of subjective, lengthy, and narrative descriptions and necessitating definitive and objective shorthand for classification of health care services.

History of coding

The history of coding for medical or dental purposes can actually be traced back to London, England, in the seventeenth century [2–4]. At that time, John Graunt developed a system of categorization of diseases, maladies, and conditions that attempted to identify the causes of death statistically and demographically for children younger than the age of 6 years. In 1893, based on Graunt's work, Dr. Jacques Bertillion developed the Bertillion Classification of the Causes of Death. His system was later revised, along with a name change to the International Classification of the Causes of Death, and has historically been considered the first edition of the *International Classification of Diseases* (ICD). This document was refined four more times until the World Health Organization (WHO) conducted a major revision in 1948 (the sixth edition). This major revision included a section on mortality and morbidity and was renamed the *Classification of Diseases, Injuries and Death*. In 1958, the seventh edition was published by the WHO, and a decade later, the eighth edition was published. The ninth revision by the WHO has resulted in the ICD-9-CM. It consists of a tabular list containing a numbered roster of the disease code numbers; an alphabetic index to the disease entries; and a classification system for surgical, diagnostic, and therapeutic procedures.

The American Medical Association (AMA) developed and published *Current Procedural Terminology* in 1966 to define surgical procedures more clearly, with limited sections on medicine, radiology, and laboratory procedures [2,5]. The second edition, which was published in 1970, included expanded terms and codes to designate diagnostic and therapeutic procedures in surgery, medicine, and the specialties. At that time, five-digit coding was introduced, replacing the former four-digit classification. In the middle to late 1970s, the third and fourth editions of the CPT code were introduced.

CPT descriptive terms and identifying codes currently serve to report medical procedures and services under public and private health insurance programs and for administrative management purposes, such as claims processing and developing guidelines for medical care review. The uniform language also is applied to medical education and research to provide a useful basis for local, regional, and national use comparisons.

Before 1986, the American Dental Association (ADA) recognized the need to report dental procedures and services accurately to third-party carriers [2,6]. To achieve uniformity, consistency, and specificity, the ADA developed the *Code on Dental Procedures and Nomenclature* (*Dental Code*). *The Current Dental Terminology*, first edition (CDT-1), which was released in 1991. The project to develop the CDT-1 began with a grant from the American Fund for Dental Health and took years to develop. It was a joint venture of general dentists and specialists. The CDT-2 was released in 1994 and included many revisions and additions. Initially, the dental coding system was a five-digit numeric system. The CDT-3 version was amended to an alpha-numeric system, with the first character of each code being the letter "D" to denote "dental system." This change was initiated based on the requirements of the Health Insurance Portability and Accountability Act (HIPAA) of 1996. Developing and maintaining the CDT is the responsibility of the Council on Dental Benefit Programs. Representatives seated on the council include members from the ADA-recognized dental specialties, the Health Care Financing Administration (HCFA), and many nationally recognized payer organizations. Although the initial plan for CDT revision was to be every 5 years, more frequent revisions were found to be necessary. The most recent version, the CDT 2007 to 2008, is now available in paper and electronic formats.

Nomenclature

Numeric and alpha-numeric

Although ICD.CM and CPT coding preceded CDT coding historically, their inclusion in this article is necessary for a complete understanding of codes and their effective use. Numeric coding merely refers to the use of numbers. This is the method used by the current ICD.9.CM and CPT coding systems for medically related communications, including billing. For instance, using the ICD.9.CM coding system, dental caries would be listed as 521.0, and using the CPT system, a biopsy of the anterior two thirds of the tongue with closure would be listed as 41112. To avoid confusion with medically related codes, the CDT system used alpha-numeric, or letter and number, codes. For instance, using the CDT system, an extraction of a single tooth, including local anesthesia, suturing if needed, and routine perioperative care, would be coded as D7120. As is illustrated, the one letter and four numbers represent 16 separate words. Thus precision, conciseness, and a savings of space and time are achieved.

Descriptors

A descriptor is merely the definition or description of the code being used in the verbiage format. For the CDT code D7241, the descriptor is "removal of impacted tooth–complete bony, with unusual surgical complications." Again, the 10 words in the descriptor are replaced by one letter and four numbers. Beyond the descriptor are further explanations of the meaning for the specific code within the code book. Again, using the example of D7241, the descriptor is followed by the following elaboration: "most or all of crown covered by bone; unusually difficult or complicated due to factors such as nerve dissection required, separate closure of maxillary sinus required or aberrant tooth position."

Symbols

Symbols are generally used in code books to alert the reader to new or revised codes or descriptors. For instance, using the CPT coding manual, a ● placed before the code number (eg, ● D0170) denotes the introduction of a new procedure code in this issue of the CPT code manual. A ▲ placed before the code number (eg, ▲ D3220) identifies a revision in the nomenclature only. Finally, a ►◄ placed before the descriptor, denotes a descriptor that has been revised since the last edition. For ICD.9.CM and CPT coding, similar symbols are used to denote new codes, changes in descriptors, and revised codes. Moreover, the ICD.9.CM and CPT coding systems use additional symbols, hollow shapes, and colored symbols to alert the user that additional information is necessary when using such codes.

Modifiers

Modifiers are not used for CDT coding; however, they are used for CPT and ICD.9.CM coding. For CPT coding, modifiers are attached to the five-number code by a hyphen to denote a comment of particular significance [5]. In the previous illustration that denoted a tongue biopsy (41112), a -51 would be added (eg, 41112-51) for multiple biopsies. If two surgeons did the biopsy, 41112-62 would be used. There are approximately 70 CPT modifiers [5].

For ICD.9.CM coding, the modifiers add specificity to the diagnosis. For instance, a facial fracture is coded as 802. A closed mandible fracture is coded as 802.2, however. At the highest level of specificity, a closed fracture of the alveolus of the mandible is coded as 802.27.

Common dental terminology codes

Common dental terminology code book use

The original intent for the CDT code book was to create an educational tool for dental practitioners and their staff. Over several years, it was modified and edited, and in 1996, the Federal Government under the HIPAA designated CDT as the nationally recognized coding system for reporting dental services [7].

Today, CDT allows for a consistent and uniform reporting mechanism of dental services to third-party payers and imparts useful billing information for the provider. Although most third-party payers require CDT coding for claims reimbursement, it is important to remember that the existence of a CDT code does not ensure that remuneration is made. Certain codes require preauthorization or predetermination or may be specifically excluded from a dental insurance plan.

Categories of common dental terminology codes

There are currently 12 different categories of service delineated in the CDT user's manual. For the sake of brevity, they are listed in Table 1 [6].

Use of common dental terminology codes for billing

The CDT code book is the most common system of coding for dental practitioners. The code book itself is broken into eight sections [7]:

Section 1, "Code on Dental Procedures and Nomenclature," is divided into 12 categories of service. Each category is further divided into commonly related dental procedures. Although the category headings may denote certain specialties, it does not preclude a general dental practitioner or dental specialist from using a particular code as long as it is within the scope of the professional's license.

The structure of the dental procedure codes includes the procedure code, the nomenclature, and the descriptor. The procedure code is a preceding five-character alpha-numeric system that begins with "D" and has a unique numeric component to distinguish each specific procedure. The nomenclature immediately follows the alpha-numeric code. This is the text naming

Table 1
Common dental terminology category of service and code series

I	Diagnostic	D0100–D0999
II	Preventive	D1000–D1999
III	Restorative	D2000–D2999
IV	Endodontics	D3000–D3999
V	Periodontics	D4000–D4999
VI	Prosthodontics, removable	D5000–D5899
VII	Maxillofacial prosthetics	D6200–D6900
VIII	Implant services	D7000–D7999
IX	Prosthodontics, fixed	D8000–D8900
X	Oral surgery	D9000–D9999
XI	Orthodontics	D5900–D5999
XII	Adjunctive general series	D6000–D6199

Data from American Dental Association. CDT 2007–2008. Chicago: ADA; 2006. p. ii.

of the procedure. The descriptor is not included for every code but can incorporate additional details or "descriptions" of the particular code. If the nomenclature indicates that the code is "by report" or "unlisted," additional supporting documentation, such as an operative report, is required.

Section 2, "Changes to the Code," includes additions and deletions. Any material that has been added to the code is noted in underlined blue text. Any portion that was deleted from a code is shown with a red strike-through. Any codes deleted in their entirety are also listed in this section with red strike-throughs.

Section 3, "Teeth Numbering and the Oral Cavity," details the Universal/National System and appends the International Standards Organization System. The Universal/National System is the form used by the ADA for the dental claim form and on standard HIPAA electronic claim transactions for dental services.

Section 4, "ADA Dental Claim Form Completion Instructions," includes instructions on how to fill out a claim form properly; use the National Provider Identifier (NPI) numbers; and relate coding for tooth numbering, tooth surface, and area of the oral cavity as used for billing purposes.

Section 5, "Questions and Answers on the Code," is also categorized by service, just as Section 1. Each question is grouped within the category to which it relates. These questions further define the intent and use for a particular code. Additions to this section are posted on the ADA's Web site [8].

Section 6, "Glossary," defines terminology used in the nomenclature or descriptor of a code. Entries are listed in alphabetic order and are defined in simplistic nonclinical terms.

Section 7, "Numeric Index to the Code," lists the codes by category of service in order. The page number on which the code and descriptor can be found is noted. This section also indicates any change in the code, noting whether it was an addition, deletion, or revision.

Section 8, "Alphabetic Index to the Code," indicates or cross-references all applicable codes in alphabetic order by term and includes page number(s) on which the code and descriptor related to the term can be found.

Current procedural terminology codes

Current procedural terminology code book use

In 2000, the Department of Health and Human Services selected the CPT code book as the national coding standard for all medical professional services and procedures under the HIPAA. For all electronic medical claim submissions, CPT coding is mandated [9,10].

Categories of current procedural terminology codes

As displayed in Table 2, there are 14 major sections of CPT codes that are based on the body system or service to be rendered [5]. They are further

Table 2
Current procedural terminology section numbers (beginning with)

Evaluation and management	99201
Anesthesiology	00100
Integumentary system	10040
Musculoskeletal system	20000
Respiratory system	30000
Cardiovascular system	33010
Digestive system	40490
Urinary system	50010
Male and female genital system	54000
Nervous system	61000
Eye and ocular adnexa	65091
Radiology	70010
Pathology and laboratory	80048
Medicine	90281

Data from Kirschner CG, Anderson CA, Beebe M, et al, editors. Current procedural terminology, CPT 2001, professional edition. Chicago: American Medical Association Press; 2001. p. 1–616.

divided into three major categories of code sets. Category I codes are most applicable to dentistry. The other categories of codes merely serve as an informational prospective from a dental medicine vantage point.

Use of current procedural terminology codes for billing

The application of category I codes for billing is reviewed in the following section [9,10].

Evaluation and management services (CPT 99201–99499)

Evaluation and management (E/M) codes are divided into three broad categories: office visits, hospital visits, and consultations. There are additional subcategories. E/M services are then classified into supplementary levels as identified by particular codes. There are three basic components to consider when determining the appropriate level of service: history, examination (Box 1), and medical decision making. Medical decision making is determined by three factors:

- The number of possible diagnoses or management options
- The volume and complexity of records, tests, or information considered
- The risk for significant complications, morbidity or mortality associated with the problem, diagnostic procedure, and management options

Anesthesia services (CPT 00100–01999, 99100–99140)

Anesthesiology codes include pre-, peri-, and postoperative care. For instance, a provider who is administering moderate conscious sedation and care of a patient would use codes 99143 through 99145. When performing moderate sedation, the following services are inclusive: assessment of the

Box 1. Evaluation and management components

- History
  - Problem focused: chief complaint, along with a brief history of the chief complaint
  - Expanded problem focused: chief complaint, brief history of the chief complaint, and review of related systems
  - Detailed: chief complaint; comprehensive history; review of complaint related systems; a limited review of additional systems; and significant past, family, or social history directly related to the current condition
  - Comprehensive: chief complaint; comprehensive history; complete review of complaint related systems; review of all remaining body systems; and complete past, family, or social history
- Examination
  - Problem focused: a limited examination of the affected area or system
  - Expanded problem focused: a limited examination of the affected area or system and a review of indicative or related system(s)
  - Detailed: an extensive examination of the affected area(s) and other indicative or related system(s)
  - Comprehensive: generalized multisystem examination or a complete examination of a single system
    - CPT defines body areas as:
      - Head, including face
      - Neck
      - Chest, including breasts and axilla
      - Abdomen
      - Genitalia, groin, buttocks
      - Back
      - Each extremity
    - CPT defines systems as:
      - Eyes
      - Ears, nose, mouth, and throat
      - Cardiovascular
      - Respiratory
      - Gastrointestinal
      - Genitourinary
      - Musculoskeletal
      - Skin
      - Neurologic
      - Psychiatric
      - Hematologic, lymphatic, or immunologic

Data from American Medical Association. CPT 2007 standard edition. Chicago: AMA, 2006. p. 1–8; and Ingenix. National fee analyzer: charge data for evaluating fees nationally. Salt Lake City (UT): Ingenix; 2006.

patient; intravenous access and management; administration of anesthetic agent(s); maintenance of the sedation; monitoring of the oxygen saturation, blood pressure, and heart rate; and recovery (not reporting time). An anesthesiology physical status modifier may be applied to the procedure code to indicate the health of a patient. These modifiers mirror the American Society of Anesthesiologists' patient physical status.

Surgical services (10021–69990)

Surgery codes are divided by systems into categories: integumentary, musculoskeletal, respiratory, cardiovascular, digestive, urinary, male/female genital, and nervous. Unless stated otherwise, the services provided by the surgeon include local anesthesia; one related E/M encounter on the day of or day before surgery; immediate postoperative care; operative report; communication with other providers, family members, and patient; writing orders; recovery evaluation; and typical postoperative follow-up.

Radiology services, including nuclear medicine and diagnostic ultrasound (70010–79999)

Radiology procedures are primarily composed of technical and professional components. The global service is reflected in the CPT code; if the same provider or facility did not carry out both components, a modifier should be used. When a provider performs only the professional component, the modifier "26" should be used. There is not a current CPT modifier for the technical component; however, payers may require the Healthcare Common Procedure Coding System (HCPCS) level II modifier "TC" to distinguish the technical component [10].

Pathology and laboratory services (80048–89356)

Pathology and laboratory procedures are often coded by what is being tested, without regard to how; however, some procedures are coded by how they are performed. It is important to identify which methodology is used for each specific code. Typically, the code represents the technical component only; however, there are particular codes that contain the technical and professional components. As mentioned previously, if a global code is used but only the professional component was rendered, a modifier "26" should be used.

In the insurance-driven health care environment, supporting documentation related to the request for pathology and laboratory services is crucial for reimbursement. The doctor ordering the test should adequately document the need for the test with proper medical coding.

Medicine services, except anesthesiology (90281–99199, 99500–99602)

Most medicine codes are for diagnostic and therapeutic services. They include the administration of vaccines, immunizations, specialty specific procedures, and certain special services. A good number of these codes are global and may require a modifier "26" if only the professional component is rendered. The coding for after-hours patient services and additional supplies provided by a physician, in addition to what is normally required for a particular service, is contained within this section.

How does this apply to dentistry?

Because the CPT coding system is used in conjunction with the ICD.9.CM coding system for submission claims, its application to dentistry is discussed in the ICD.9.CM subsection entitled "How does this apply to dentistry," to avoid redundancy.

International Classification of Diseases, Ninth Revision, Clinical Modification

International Classification of Diseases, Ninth Revision, Clinical Modification code book use

Although ICD.9.CM codes were designed to provide a uniform classification system for the purposes of education and research, they are more commonly used today for "medical necessity" determinations related to procedures performed. They complement CPT codes in that CPT codes provide the procedure and service information and ICD.9.CM codes provide the reason or rationale for a particular procedure or service. Since 1989 in the United States, doctors are required by law to submit ICD.9.CM coding for any reimbursement from Medicare and Medicaid Services. Additionally, most third-party payers require ICD.9.CM coding for any medical procedure performed [11].

Category of International Classification of Diseases, Ninth Revision, Clinical Modification codes

The core of the ICD.9.CM system of coding actually has 17 separate categories of codes (Table 3) that categorize a disease or injury based mostly on the body system involved or the etiology [3,4]. E codes, V codes, and M codes can be included in this system. The E codes are based on external (thus, the E) cause of injury or poisoning, V codes are based on other factors influencing health status and contact with health services, and M codes are based on the morphology (thus, the M) of a neoplasm. These supplemental ICD.9.CM coding systems are beyond the scope of this article [3,4].

Use of International Classification of Diseases, Ninth Revision, Clinical Modification codes for billing

In order to code ICD.9.CM correctly, it is necessary to determine the reason for the encounter. Suspected conditions and "rule-out" diagnoses cannot be coded. It is important that a correctly identified diagnosis is reported.

When a diagnosis has not been established, it is appropriate to indicate symptoms and conditions; however, if a specific diagnosis is established, the code that most appropriately represents the patient's condition should be used. For inpatient care, a "primary" diagnosis is established and additional noninherent conditions of the primary diagnosis are also listed. For outpatient care, the most relevant diagnosis is reported as the "first listed." Additional germane conditions are also reported. For inpatient and outpatient care, chronic conditions should be indicated if they are relevant to the condition and treatment of the patient [11].

The ICD.9.CM code book is divided into two major sections: the index and the table. It is important first to locate the condition in the index. The index is an alphabetic listing of diseases, conditions, signs, and symptoms with a corresponding diagnosis code. The tabular section is organized in code order, with each subsection containing the three-digit "generic" code heading and the subheading expanded to include fourth, and sometimes fifth, digit extensions. Often, beginning in the tabular section can result in a less specific or inaccurate diagnosis; however, it is necessary to consult the tables to assign certain conditions to the diagnosis necessary for complete and accurate coding.

Most codes require a fourth digit. Moreover, many codes require an additional fifth digit extension. These extensions are used to provide additional diagnostic information or information related to state of the patient or the specific area affected. If the same fifth digit classification is to be used for an entire category, it should be noted at the beginning of the category. The fourth and fifth digit extensions are separated from the primary code by a decimal point.

How does this apply to dentistry?

Medical procedures routinely performed by dentists include trauma, biopsies, and dental treatment as a result of or in anticipation of a cancer-related treatment. Additionally, the overall health of a patient may require that routine dental treatment be performed in an acute care facility. As a result, most care facilities require that the provider submit all necessary third-party CPT and ICD.9.CM preauthorization applications for treatment at such facilities. Thus, it is important that the dental care provider has a basic understanding of the CPT and ICD.9.CM classification system (see Table 3) so that he or she can acquire third-party authorization for these services.

Billing

For the purposes of financial transactions, specifically dental billing, patients may be categorized as private pay or insured. The private pay classification includes not only those patients maintaining no third-party insurance coverage but those patients maintaining coverage with no

Table 3
ICD.9.CM coding guidelines

Category of disease or injury of body system	ICD.9.CM numeric code range	Application and significance to dentistry
Infectious diseases and parasitic diseases	001.0–139.0	It is important for the dental provider to understand that HIV infections can only be coded in cases in which the disease has been confirmed; however, if the patient indicates an HIV-positive status, the disease status is considered conclusive and no additional serology is required.
Neoplasms	140.0–239.0	It is not always possible to provide a complete diagnosis at the time of treatment, particularly in an outpatient setting. This is a common quandary for the dental provider diagnosing a neoplasm. Often, at the initial examination and excision, a definitive diagnosis is not ascertainable. A pathologist may be required to render a confirmative or negative opinion. As such, neoplasm coding should be rendered based on the course of treatment directed. If a dental practitioner diagnoses a benign neoplasm and follow-up care is directed toward this outcome, the diagnosis should be coded in accordance. If it is anticipated that the neoplasm is malignant and follow-up care is aimed at such, it should be coded as malignant. If a practitioner is uncertain of the etiology of the neoplasm, and follow-up care is reflective, the diagnosis should indicate uncertain.
Endocrine, nutritional, and metabolic diseases and immunity disorders	240.0–279.0	If the type of diabetes mellitus is not indicated, it is assumed to be type II. All diabetic disorders require an additional fifth digit that reflects whether the condition is controlled or uncontrolled.
Diseases of blood and blood-forming organs	280.0–289.0	For the dental provider it is important to note that patients who have various clotting disorders may require routine dental extractions or other invasive treatment in an acute medical facility. For such treatment to be approved or reimbursed by third-party payers, proper coding of such diseases is necessary. As well, if partial thromboplastin time and prothrombin time laboratory tests are indicated, all necessary related conditions should be coded to avoid medical necessity edits.
Mental disorders	290.0–319.0	Many patients who have acute mental illness may not tolerate simple dental procedures without deep sedation. Also, patients who have a documented severe phobia related to dental treatment may require deep sedation. Often, it is necessary to provide care for these individuals in an acute care setting. For such treatment to be approved or reimbursed by third-party payers, proper coding of such disorders is necessary.

Diseases of nervous systems and sense organs	320.0–389.0	Notable for the dental professional in this section is that it includes trigeminal nerve disorders and facial and cranial nerve disorders.
Diseases of circulatory system	390.0–459.0	Significant for the provider is that if a patient does not have a documented history of hypertension and has an elevated blood pressure reading, the appropriate diagnosis of "hypertension, transient" (ICD.9.CM: 796.2) should be assigned.
Diseases of respiratory system	460.0–519.0	Chronic airway obstruction is a nonspecific code that should not be used unless the provider is unable to ascertain the type of chronic obstructive pulmonary disease or asthma affecting the patient.
Diseases of digestive system	520.0–579.0	This section is by far the most frequently used by the dental provider and includes diseases of the oral cavity, salivary glands, and jaws. It details disorders of tooth development and eruption, supernumerary teeth, and disturbances in tooth formation and structure. It classifies dental caries, excessive attrition, abrasion, erosion, pathologic resorption, ankylosis, pulp disorders, periodontitis, abscesses, and many other dental alveolar disorders. Cystic and inflammatory conditions and dentofacial anomalies and abnormalities are also contained within this section. Most notably, unlike most trauma injury codes, which are listed from 800 to 999.9, loss of teeth attributable to trauma is included within this section.
Diseases of genitourinary system	580.0–629.0	Most of this section does not relate to conditions necessarily coded by the dental care provider. The most notable items are for patients who have end-stage renal disease or status post-kidney transplant, because these conditions may necessitate treatment rendered in an acute health care facility.
Complications of pregnancy, childbirth and the puerperium	630.0–677.0	This section is not of much significance for the dental care provider.
Diseases of skin and subcutaneous tissue	680.0–709.0	Coding for cellulitis and abscesses, including the face, are contained within this section in addition to keloid scaring and other hypertrophic and atrophic conditions of the skin.
Diseases of musculoskeletal and connective tissue	710.0–739.0	This section contains pertinent coding information detailing osteopathies, chondropathies, and acquired musculoskeletal deformities. For the dental care provider, it is relevant to mention that osteomyelitis of the jaw is specifically excluded under this section and is housed with diseases of the digestive system (ICD.9.CM: 526.4 or 526.5).

(*continued on next page*)

Table 3 (*continued*)

Category of disease or injury of body system	ICD.9.CM numeric code range	Application and significance to dentistry
Congenital anomalies	740.0–759.0	Of note, when documenting an anomaly as a secondary condition, it is not necessary to code additional conditions that are present as inherent components of the anomaly.
Newborn guidelines	760.0–779.0	This section does not normally relate to the dental care provider, with the possible exception of birth trauma that requires oral and maxillofacial surgery intervention.
Signs, symptoms, and ill-defined conditions	780.0–799.0	This section is specifically designed for the practitioner to document conditions and symptoms that are transient or have an unknown etiology. Common use for the dental care provider may include syncope, dizziness, pallor, flushing, nausea, or abnormal blood pressure readings without specific diagnosis.
Injury and poisoning	800.0–999.0	For dental providers, medical billing is often necessary for trauma-related procedures. When coding multiple unilateral or bilateral fractures of the same bone, use fourth digit subcategories and code each fracture uniquely by specific site.

Data from Baierschmidt C, Ericson B, Miller S, et al, editors. Physician ICD.9.CM, vols. 1 and 2. Salt Lake City (UT): Medicode Publications; 1999; and Hart AC, Ford B, editors. ICD.9.CM professional, for physicians, international classification of diseases, 9th revision, clinical modification, vols. 1 and 2. Salt Lake City (UT): Ingenix Publications; 2007.

reimbursement for the intended services, specifically patients with medical insurance only and those with policy exclusions for some or all dental services. Accurate and complete capture of any and all available insurance information as presented by the patient is requisite but should also be accompanied by independent verification directly with the carrier, whenever possible. Verification of insurance coverage before dental treatment allows the practitioner and the patient to be adequately prepared for the monetary aspects related to receipt of care. Also, disclosing the financial responsibility to each patient allows the patient to provide informed consent for care he or she is about to receive.

Medicare

Since the inception of Medicare in 1965, dental services have been excluded. Section 1862 [42 U.S.C. 1395y] (a) (12) of the Social Security Act cites the exclusion to dental services as follows [12]:

> where such expenses are for services in connection with the care, treatment, filling, removal or replacement of teeth or structures directly supporting teeth, except that payment may be made under Part A in the case of inpatient hospital services in connection with the provision of such dental services if the individual, because of his underlying medical condition and clinical status or because of the severity of the dental procedure, requires hospitalization in connection with the provision of such services.

There are two local medical review policies (LMRPs) and one national coverage determination (NCD) that further define when services may or may not be covered. To summarize the policies and determinations, Medicare only covers dental care for prehead and neck radiation therapy to treat neoplastic diseases, an examination as part of a comprehensive transplant workup, treatment related to a traumatic injury to the facial structures, and other treatment related to a cancer diagnosis. The Center for Medicare and Medicaid Services offers a complete listing of the service limitations and guidelines on their Web site [13].

Medicaid

Medicaid programs, established by Title XIX of the Social Security Act, provide state-sponsored financial guarantorship for health care services rendered to qualifying low-income individuals or those with disabilities or other health conditions [14]. These programs work in a manner similar to a commercial insurance plan with coverage exclusions and frequency limitations. Each state independently determines the coverage and eligibility protocol for Medicaid recipients with permanent addresses in that state. In general, Medicaid covers routine and preventive care for recipients but may provide specialty care for children or for those with special health care needs, including concomitant medical conditions. For additional information regarding Medicaid programs for the individual states, contact the Department for

Health and Family Services or related authority within the state or commonwealth.

Third-party coverage

Many employers choose to offer third-party commercial dental insurance coverage for their full-time employees. Coverage may be issued in the form of a dental rider for preventive services attached to an existing medical insurance plan or as a distinct policy underwritten by a carrier independent of medical coverage. Most commercial dental plans offer comprehensive coverage for routine and preventative dental services, such as examinations, prophylaxis, and fluoride treatments for children, with frequency limitations on a plan or calendar-year basis. Coverage for restorative dental work and specialty services is generally limited to 30% to 80% and often includes an annual deductible amount that must be satisfied before commencement of coverage.

Commercial third-party carriers often seek to enter into contractual agreements with dental providers, exchanging accessibility to covered lives for a financial discount of covered services. Contracts with commercial carriers are negotiable, but the carriers commonly seek a 20% to 50% discount of the dental provider's usual and customary fee (UCF). These contracts may also include provisions binding the provider to seek remuneration only from the carrier for covered services and prohibit "balance" billing of the patient for amounts discounted. Many contracts also include a specified time frame for submitting claims, know as "timely filing," after which the claim is denied by the carrier with a prohibition against collection from the patient.

Third-party commercial insurance contracts encourage patient referrals by listing contracted dental providers, commonly known as "participating providers," in a directory used by patients for choosing health care services. These listings are valuable for building business, but the advantage should always be weighed against the administrative burden of the contract for the dental office.

Self-pay

The patient classified as private pay should be made aware of potential financial responsibility as early as practical within the treatment process. A legal statement consenting to the acceptance of financial responsibility should be read and signed by the patient, legal guardian, or power of attorney, as applicable, before any financial responsibility is incurred and should include the signature of a witness. A statement of financial responsibility need not contain specific information about treatment or finite cost estimates but should indicate that treatment plans and cost estimates are "best guesses" and may be subject to change at the discretion of the provider. The party accepting the financial responsibility may then be added to the patient's record as a guarantor.

Developing a clear, concise, and enforceable written payment policy ensures equitable management for all patients, insured and noninsured. Payment policies should be displayed and made accessible for reference by office staff and patients, establishing consistent application regarding expectation for payment appropriate to the level of care. In addition, payment policies should clearly define the terms of any financial agreement and delineate by type of service when payment is expected in advance of or at the time of service and when payment may be delayed or made over an extended period. Key items for inclusion in the payment policy are the percentage of the total amount due for each type of service, the associated timeline for payment of that percentage, an explanation of any calculation involved in determining any minimum payment for amounts financed over multiple payment periods, and penalties for late or missed payments or failure to honor the agreement as written. Payment policies should also include information related to any available recourse should an inability to pay arise. Payment policies must applied fairly and reliably for private pay patients and insured patients, with deductibles, copayments, coinsurance, or other patient financial responsibility as determined by the carrier.

For those patients receiving services that require repayment terms, a legal document detailing the terms of the financial arrangement should be agreed on and delivered in writing for the guarantor's signature before the commencement of treatment. Adherence to the Truth in Lending Consumer Credit Cost Disclosure Act is mandatory for any account with balances payable in four or more installments [15], but operational economies may be recognized by following the guidelines of this regulation for all installment accounts. The act requires full disclosure of the total balance, the number of payments, the amount of each payment, and any applicable interest rates or charges (including a rate of 0.00%) [15]. It is also recommended that the financial contract include a statement explaining to the patient that the payment arrangements are based on treatment estimates and may require renegotiation should treatment options be revised or amended.

Paper

Dental services may be billed to most third-party dental benefit plans, commercial and governmental, using a paper version of the standardized ADA-approved claim form. There are currently four paper versions of the ADA claim form: 1994, 2000, 2002, and 2006. The ADA supports the use of the most current form [16], but carriers often have specific requirements and may request an alternate version of the form. Comprehensive instructions for the proper completion of the ADA 2006 form may be found in the ADA Publication entitled *CDT 2007/2008*.

Timely and consistent submission of paper claims for services rendered by the dental office maintains a regular and predictable cash flow to the practice from third-party payers. Processing time for paper claims by insurers includes time necessary for data entry from the paper form into a claims payment system, eligibility and service review, claim adjudication, and deployment of a remittance instrument, most often in the form of a check or direct deposit. Turn-around time for payment of claims submitted using the paper form must be calculated in consideration of mail and processing time and generally exceeds 30 calendar days.

At the present time, methods for submitting attachments to claims, such as radiography and operative reports, are limited to hard-copy submissions. It is advisable to submit claims requiring supporting documentation for consideration of reimbursement on paper with the documentation attached to avoid unnecessary delays attributable to lost, misdirected, or mismatched information. An alternative process, which is significantly less reliable, calls for electronic submission of the claim with subsequent hard-copy supporting documentation being mailed to the payer for match at the payer site.

Electronic

As computer technology advanced during the 1990s, the personal computer became ubiquitous in the health care and dental office setting, creating opportunities to increase the efficiency of the historically paper-based process of claims submission. Electronic methods of submitting claims by means of carrier Web sites or through national claims clearinghouses have distinct advantages over traditional paper methods of submission, including reduced turn-around time because of elimination of mail time and data entry lags at the carrier site.

The HIPAA of 1996 under Title II mandated the development and acceptance of a single and universal electronic format for electronic claims [17]. For dentistry, this is the "837D" transaction. Adoption of this single format has clarified the process for individual providers by requiring that all carriers accept the same file type and eliminating the need for carrier-specific or proprietary formats.

Most popular electronic claim submission software programs include a routine list of claim edits, displaying and notating claims that do not pass the initial demographic and data element protocol. Showing these edits and any subsequent rejections permits real-time correction of erroneous data elements, allowing the health care or dental provider to correct such items as incorrect policy numbers, dates of birth, subscriber demographic data, or coding errors immediately, thus eliminating the delay associated with paper filing and associated carrier rejections.

Data clearinghouses for electronic claim submission offer three levels of reports for follow-up on submitted claims. A first-level rejection report should be received from the clearinghouse within 24 hours of submission. This report details those items not passing the initial carrier edits, such as provider contract not found, provider license number miss-match, or patient not found. Forty-eight hours from submission, the submitting provider should be able to access a second-level confirmation report acknowledging the receipt of submitted claims by the carrier. This confirmation report may also include status indicators, such as claim pending review, claim adjudicated, or claim approved for payment. Within 3 business days, the third-level rejection report should be received showing coverage exclusions and cancelled policies.

National provider identification number use

In addition to the standardization of electronic formats, standardization of health care transactions under the HIPAA has also included the introduction of the National Provider Identifier (NPI) system. The NPI is designed to replace all previous (legacy) provider identifiers, including the UPIN (Universal Provider Identification Number) and carrier-specific "provider numbers." Individual health care and dental providers (type 1) and health care groups and facilities (type 2) are assigned a single 10-digit NPI number. The deadline for NPI use was originally May 23, 2007, but it has subsequently been altered to May 23, 2008 for small health plans [18].

All health care and dental providers billing third-party commercial and governmental payers should apply for an NPI. NPI assignment is completed through the National Plan and Provider Enumeration System (NPPES), which may be accessed on-line [19].

Summary

With technologic advances and increased awareness and consumption of health care, especially dental care, the cost of health care has dramatically increased over the past century. General dentists and specialists are offering and providing diverse and more complex treatment procedures for their patient population. These patients have some form of third-party dental or medical insurance that covers a certain percentage of their treatment, or they have no insurance and are responsible for the entire cost of care they receive.

Numeric and alpha-numeric coding and classification protocols permit successful interaction of health care providers with one another and with third-party payers. Specifically, coding permits an effective and consistent means of communicating accurate yet concise accounts of services rendered. Coding and classifications systems have evolved over the past several decades through edits, modifications, and refinements, producing a nationally recognized system of numeric and alpha-numeric codes, specifically ICD.9.CM, CPT, and CDT. It is of great importance for health care providers to understand the application of these codes, because incomplete or incorrect use of codes could mean a refusal or delayed reimbursement. Several and simultaneous incidents of refusal or delayed reimbursement can have a significant impact on the cash flow and, in some cases, can be detrimental to the viability of a health care setting, especially a newly emerging one.

CDT codes are most commonly used by the dental professional; as of 1996, under the HIPAA, they are designated as the nationally recognized coding system for reporting dental services in the United States. Conversely, CPT and ICD.9.CM codes are more commonly used by physicians. These two coding systems complement each other (ie, whereas CPT coding provides the procedure and service information, ICD.9.CM coding provides the reason or rationale for a particular procedure or service). These codes are more commonly used for "medical necessity" determinations. General dentists and specialists who routinely perform care, including trauma-related care, biopsies, and dental treatment as a result of or in anticipation of a cancer-related treatment, are likely to use these codes.

Most claims for services provided can be submitted by means of paper forms or electronically, with electronic submission having the advantage of reduced turn-around time because of elimination of mail time and data entry lags at the carrier site.

References

[1] American Medical Billing Association Online. Electronic claims processing facts. Claims transit. Available at: http://www.webcom.com/medical/elec_clm.htm. Accessed May 14, 2007.

[2] Haug RH, Allaire M, Trangoni K, et al, editors. Parameters and pathway: clinical practice guidelines for oral and maxillofacial surgery. Chicago: American Association of Oral and Maxillofacial Surgeons; 2001.

[3] Baierschmidt C, Ericson B, Miller S, et al, editors. Physician ICD.9.CM, vols. 1 and 2. Salt Lake City (UT): Medicode Publications; 1999.

[4] Hart AC, Ford B, editors. ICD.9.CM professional, for physicians, international classification of diseases, 9th revision, clinical modification, vols. 1 and 2. Salt Lake City (UT): Ingenix Publications; 2007.

[5] Kirschner CG, Anderson CA, Beebe M, et al, editors. Current procedural terminology, CPT 2001, professional edition. Chicago: American Medical Association Press; 2001.

[6] Current dental terminology, CDT 3, users manual. Chicago: American Dental Association Press; 2000.

[7] American Dental Association. CDT 2007–2008. Chicago: ADA; 2006.

[8] American Dental Association. Available at: http://www.ada.org/goto/dentalcode.

[9] American Medical Association. CPT® 2007 standard edition. Chicago: AMA; 2006.

[10] Ingenix. National fee analyzer: charge data for evaluating fees nationally. Salt Lake City (UT): Ingenix; 2006.

[11] Hart A, Hopkins C. ICD-9-CM professional: for physicians, vols. 1 and 2. Salt Lake City (UT): Ingenix; 2006.

[12] Social Security Online. Exclusions from coverage and Medicare as secondary payer. Available at: http://www.ssa.gov/op_home/ssact/title18/1862.htm. Accessed August 24, 2007.

[13] Centers for Medicare and Medicaid Services. Available at: www.cms.hhs.gov/MedicareDentalCoverage/.

[14] Social Security Online. Title XIX—grants to states for medical assistance programs. Available at: http://www.ssa.gov/op_home/ssact/title19/1900.htm. Accessed August 23, 2007.

[15] Robinson-Crowley Christine. Understanding patient financial services. Gaithersburg (MD): Aspen Publishers, Inc; 1997.

[16] American Dental Association Online. ADA dental claim form. Available at: http://www.ada.org/prof/resources/topics/claimform.asp. Accessed July 30, 2007.

[17] Centers for Medicaid and Medicare Services Online. HIPAA—general information. December 2005. Available at: http://www.cms.hhs.gov/hipaageninfo/. Accessed August 17, 2007.
[18] Centers for Medicaid and Medicare Services Online. Regulations and guidance/HIPAA administrative simplification/national provider identifier standard. January 2004. Available at: http://questions.cms.hhs.gov/cgi-bin/cmshhs.cfg. Accessed August 17, 2007.
[19] Available at: www.nppes.cms.hhs.gov.

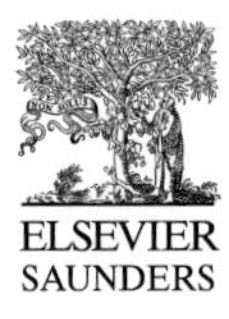

THE DENTAL CLINICS OF NORTH AMERICA

Dent Clin N Am 52 (2008) 529–534

Basic Bookkeeping and Avoiding Theft

Ian M. Nelson, CPA, LLC

3 Cornell St, West Orange, NJ 07052, USA

Basic bookkeeping as defined by licensed professionals and veteran bookkeepers or accountants provides a bright line area of subtle differences among the practices of many dentists. These differences, when seen from the viewpoint of a medical professional, are sometimes startlingly different than that of a veteran accountant or bookkeeper. What, then, is bookkeeping? Bookkeeping is the art of meticulously recording all the transactions of any business enterprise and consolidating them in a certain way, typically by type. It is defined by *Webster's* dictionary as "the detailed recording of a company's transactions such as its sales and expenses." This article examines how practitioners interpret and implement their role as bookkeepers and discusses controls, appropriate documentation, and theft prevention.

Many beginning dental practitioners focus on collecting fees and paying bills; they record these transactions in a checkbook. Most fees are collected after patients are treated, and the fees range from deductibles, insurance billings, or full collection. Patients are sometimes assisted in filing insurance claims. Recently, many practitioners have developed creditor relationships that can facilitate quicker payments.

When opening a practice, practitioners often choose accounting software which allows them to bill an insurance company effectively. However, little coordination may exist between accounts receivable and their bill payment system, the result of which can be devastating.

Some practitioners employ a "one-write system" that allows them to document their transactions while paying their bills. This system is quite effective for recording expenses. It also allows for a classification of expenses and a simultaneous balancing of the practitioner's checkbook. However, the summarization of these transactions requires tedious steps because the process is manual and each expense must be grouped (ie, classified) and totaled. Deposits may be summarized from the one-write sheets or check stubs, but

E-mail address: ian.cpa@gmail.com

0011-8532/08/$ - see front matter
doi:10.1016/j.cden.2008.02.004 **dental.theclinics.com**

the details affecting each patient must be recorded in a sub-ledger to ensure accuracy. In addition, the practitioner must adjust patient ledgers to reflect any discounts or similar adjustments. This process is susceptible to human error such as omissions and arithmetic errors.

The practitioner must also repeat identical procedures to record unpaid and paid bills. This is called the accounts payable system. Because numbers will have to be transferred to sub-ledgers for all suppliers, errors of omission, transpositions, and other related issues are likely to occur. The practitioner must also reconcile the checkbook. During reconciliation, in-house records are compared to bank records to ensure accuracy; all paid checks and collected funds are accounted for.

Because of the demanding nature of most manual accounting systems, the practitioner should choose software that does the following: records patient treatments via defined diagnostic codes; records transactions affecting accounts receivables and accounts payable; records cash transactions; simplifies summarization of data; and provides thorough reporting of all activity within the practice. Crucially, a summary of a patient's history shows which vital services were rendered and when.

The art of recording transactions and "theft-proofing" one's business requires every business owner to establish a system of controls. These controls are activated any time a transaction is recorded, changed or deleted. Importantly, these controls reveal if someone fails to perform any important steps. Professional accountants call this system of "checks and balances" internal controls.

A system of internal controls requires every practitioner to know the process by which transactions are initiated and recorded. The process encompasses fees for service, bill paying, and governmental compliance. Fees for service and bill paying can be managed completely in-house. Governmental compliance is started in-house, but it is reviewed at its end point by a governmental employee. Compliance is created through a payroll reporting and requires each employer to remit funds to the government regularly. In addition, extensive reporting must comply with the law to avoid a serious negative impact. The serious impact could include but is not limited to penalties, fines, interest, and other punitive mandates created by statute. Payroll itself can present problems for employers because of internal control weaknesses, (ie, unsupervised employees), inflation of hours, rate changes, and the creation of phantom employees.

Employee negligence in processing and remitting payroll liabilities can cause excessive penalties and interests. Accordingly, an outside payroll service, such as Paychex or ADP is recommended. However, before submitting time sheets to the payroll company, the manager should ascertain that all hourly, per diem, and salaried employees have accurately recorded their time. The manager should signify approval by their signature. Contact with the payroll company should be limited to authorized persons only. This limits any manipulation of the payroll.

All companies are required to file quarterly reports with federal and state authorities. Failure to comply can cause a business to be shut down. The primary system of checks and balances that fights employee theft begins with appropriate intervention and a state of mind. In designing and developing a system of internal controls, critical areas of operation are examined. In a dental practice, these areas are: fees for service; fee collection; cash management; bill paying; and payroll expenses. In managing the fee for service function, office personnel must have the ability to identify the patients treated and the collections made from them.

In addition, immediate control must be established over all daily cash collections. In small dental practices, the practitioner may be the most likely person to do this. In larger practices, an office manager usually assumes this role. In order to maintain tight control over cash, verification of daily collections must be done and deposits made regularly. All deposits must be verified by a second person; this minimizes any misappropriation. After daily collections are verified and deposited, the bookkeeper must record all amounts to update patient ledgers. The office manager or the dental practitioner should review patient accounts to ensure that they are updated. This step not only simplifies the collection process, but any "unrecorded" collections can be identified.

Many offices maintain a petty cash account that is used for emergency needs of the office. Withdrawal of petty cash funds should be authorized at the highest level possible. Each disbursement should be documented with a prenumbered receipt that is signed by the person receiving cash. The recipient should be required to submit a third party receipt for all funds being reimbursed.

For offices that use metered postage, an office manager should be required to validate postage needs before authorizing any distribution. Because a postage meter can be subject to unauthorized use, a key or password control should be employed. Several vendors, such as Pitney Bowes, typically lease postal meters and related equipment.

Also, the ordering of office supplies should be authorized and supervised by an office manager or the dental practitioner. This prevents or minimizes pilferage and abuse. Similarly, depending on its size or its frequency of use, certain items should be periodically inventoried. This allows the office to gauge usage and minimize pilferage. Some very large items may even be tagged with a control number to minimize theft of physical assets. Portable computers should be kept under lock and key.

Bill paying, like cash collection and petty cash, must be controlled to avoid a long term negative impact. All paid invoices must be voided to prevent duplication. Invoices must be reviewed for content and approved before being paid. Then, the dental practitioner can be assured that the purchases are valid.

A purchase order system should be in place to document the legitimacy of purchases. Purchase orders are used to streamline requisitioning of supplies and identify the person making the requests. All delivered products should come to an authorized person who is responsible for distribution. Receipt must be confirmed by someone's signature on the delivery invoice. Purchase orders must be signed by the office manager or the dental practitioner. Any deviation from this system could result in pilferage of supplies.

If electronic payments are used (ie, online payment), password control must also be maintained at all times. Electronic payments and credit cards have become the more popular ways to efficiently pay bills. Company credit cards should be used only by those whose judgment can be trusted and, statements should be periodically reviewed and the dental practitioner apprised of all transactions. The review can be done by a consulting accountant. Also, payment must never be made against a statement, only against original invoices. One of the most effective methods of monitoring check disbursements, electronic payments, and credit card disbursements is through bank statement reconciliations.

Bank reconciliations must be periodically reviewed by an independent accountant. Cancelled checks should always be reviewed for double endorsements that could indicate questionable or irregular business practices.

In many small practices, all bookkeeping and related functions are executed by one person. Invariably, there are the stories about a dedicated bookkeeper who never took vacation, but who is then being prosecuted for embezzlement. It is imperative that the bookkeeper take their vacation when scheduled. In addition, the bookkeeper's work should always be reviewed by an independent CPA to ensure irregularities are minimized or eliminated.

In addition to reviewing the bookkeeper's work, dental practitioners should invest in easy-to-use software which effectively captures the entire recording and reporting function. Accounting software makes the recording of routine transactions efficient. The software should have an audit trail which would identify any unauthorized charges. Also, the software should enable good reporting and enhance the quality of frequent analytical reviews.

Whereas a bookkeeping system will probably never be "just basic," its effectiveness will be based on its ability to make every transaction transparent as well as to preclude recording and concealing a fraudulent event. There is no solution for collusion; however, a system that includes timely intervention, as well as enough checks and balances, will ultimately strengthen a business.

How should a basic bookkeeping system be designed to minimize or prevent theft? The answer is: logically. Most accounting systems allow for the initial transaction to be recorded and then document the process to closure. Accordingly, any such system for a dental practice must encompass the following: initial office visits, treatment plan, payment method(s), collections, treatment plan enhancements, and follow-up documentation.

Modern technology allows dentists to transmit radiographs to an insurance agency almost immediately. In addition, unless an immediate clinical need is established during the first visit, a typical procedure requires that a patient start their soft tissue management. This is accomplished by having the hygienist or the dentist clean the patient's teeth and take radiographs. At this time, a practitioner identifies the clinical needs of the patient. This process is called the treatment plan development.

Any software used by a dental practitioner should allow setting up such plans and enable a practitioner to track all billings. Because dentistry now includes much more than fillings, any treatment software should contain diagnosis/treatment codes to facilitate the efficient billing of all services.

The accounting software enhances the practitioner's ability to reconcile services rendered and the receivable daily. In addition, the ability to routinely track one's billing allows for better monitoring of receivables, ensures timely updating of customer ledgers, and facilitates a smooth collection process. To further illustrate how internal controls help to prevent or minimize employee theft, a nearly perfect scenario is described below.

1. The front desk schedules all patients.
2. The dentist or the dental hygienist takes full mouth radiographs and does a cleaning. A chair camera can be used to remit immediately to an insurance carrier.
3. After services are rendered, the collections clerk collects the fee stipulated from the standard billing chart and the appointment clerk schedules future appointments.
4. Patient chart is reviewed and signed by the doctor, who also verifies the services to be billed for.
5. The office manager reviews the appointment schedule at day's end and compares services rendered to collections and insurance charges. A day sheet is signed by the manager to confirm accuracy and completeness.
6. Cash and check collections are summarized and sealed in an envelope after being double-verified by the manager and collection clerk.
7. The manager forwards the summarized day sheet and all collections to either the practitioner or a senior employee with responsibility for banking operations.
8. The practitioner or the senior employee responsible for banking operations prepares the day's deposit. This person confirms the totals, signs the day sheet, and forwards same to the bookkeeper.
9. The bookkeeper updates the patient records.
10. The receivables are monitored by the collections clerk to facilitate timely collection.
11. An independent accountant is used to review and test transactions to ensure proper recording.

Although the above scenario describes a process managed by multiple employees, it underscores the practitioner's need to cover many critical functions with limited staff. It is also a reminder as to why a practitioner must know what is occurring in the practice.

Avoiding theft is the ultimate goal. The creation of the right process provides quality results and helps good employees remain motivated. When screening employees, a background check may include fingerprinting and a search for a criminal record. Key employees who have control over cash should also be bonded. Bonding takes place after all background checks have been completed and the prospective employee's record is clear. Bonding can be approved by insurance or surety companies.

After employees are screened, tested for alcohol or drug abuse, and fingerprinted, they should have their job descriptions presented to them. In addition, their compensation should be competitive with market rates. This allows an employee to feel employer loyalty, to feel confident based on their defined role, and to be a part of a quality practice.

The office manager should consistently prepare employee schedules to maintain consistency and a sense of orderliness. All hourly employees must have their time sheets reviewed and approved by a person at least two levels above them. Detailed attention must be given to days off, vacations, and personal time, as well as hourly rates. Unapproved overtime and inflated hourly rates can devastate a business; therefore, salaried employees should be utilized as much as possible.

In safeguarding the financial aspects of a dental practice, internal controls may rely heavily on the dental practitioner themselves or on the most trusted personnel. Effective control is achieved when no assumptions are made and when most, if not all, items are questioned by the dentist. Personal involvement is a must for all dental practitioners if they are to maintain order in their practice, prevent theft, and keep costs under control.

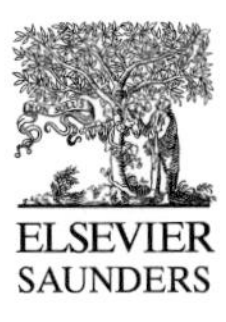
ELSEVIER
SAUNDERS

Dent Clin N Am 52 (2008) 535–547

THE DENTAL CLINICS OF NORTH AMERICA

Employee Relations

Eric T.K. Demann, DMD[a,*], Pamela S. Stein, DMD[b], Christine Levitt[c], Keith E. Shelton, MPA[d]

[a]*University of Kentucky, College of Dentistry, Kentucky Clinic Dentistry, A-219, Lexington, KY 40536-0284, USA*
[b]*University of Kentucky, College of Medicine, 800 Rose Street, MN 210, Lexington, KY 40536-0298, USA*
[c]*Office of Administrative Affairs, University of Kentucky, College of Dentistry, 800 Rose Street, D-131, Lexington, KY 40536-0297, USA*
[d]*University of Kentucky, College of Dentistry, 800 Rose Street, M-128, Lexington, KY 40536-0297, USA*

The face of employee relations has changed a great deal in the practice of dentistry. Several years ago, a dentist may have had only one staff member who answered the phone, made appointments, and assisted at the chair. This situation is a stark contrast to the dentist of today who may have 20 or more employees on his or her dental team. From insurance specialists to scheduling coordinators, the staff has expanded and become more specialized to improve the efficiency and productivity of the individual employee and the practice as a whole.

No dentist could argue the value of a pleasant, competent, and reliable staff. Hiring and retaining excellent employees in the dental office is integral to the success of the practice; however, managing a staff of several employees can be challenging. This article attempts to assist the dentist in this regard by discussing some of the most pertinent human relation topics in the practice of dentistry.

Recruitment

When starting a new dental practice, expanding an existing practice, or replacing someone who has left, there are several aspects to consider before hiring a new employee. Some of these aspects are establishing job expectations, advertising, interviewing, and pre-employment credentialing of applicants [1].

* Corresponding author.
E-mail address: edemann@yahoo.com (E.T.K. Demann).

doi:10.1016/j.cden.2008.02.005

Job expectations

A job description should be written that clearly communicates job expectations and the type of person needed for the job. The job description should include specific job duties, skills required to perform the job, physical attributes an employee must have to perform the duties (eg, the ability to lift heavy objects or sit for long periods of time), credentials, an acceptable education level, and experience necessary for employment [2]. The description should incorporate the practice philosophy or mission and how the employee will fit into the big picture. In addition, a statement should be added that articulates compliance with local, state, and federal laws [3].

After the job description has been written, it is time to begin recruiting. Having a happy and successful team of employees can be an inexpensive and effective recruitment tool. Open positions or soon-to-be vacancies may be communicated to internal employees so they can be on the lookout for potential candidates in their network of friends and associates. A dentist's social, professional, or academic colleagues may also aid in recruitment.

Advertising

If advertising is necessary, a budget should be determined beforehand and appropriate publications for advertisements selected [4]. Hourly positions such as dental assistants, dental hygienists, receptionists, and business managers may be advertised in local newspapers and online job postings. When recruiting a dentist, particularly someone with a specialty degree, it may be necessary to advertise regionally or even nationally. Journals, dental schools, state dental associations, and specialized online publications are a good way to advertise for dentists. The advertisements should reach a diverse population [4].

Because the advertisement should spark interest and create a positive first impression in potential applicants, it should be constructed carefully and thoughtfully. It may be helpful to talk to existing employees and find out what attracted them to the practice, incorporating that information into the advertisement [4]. For example, the training provided, flexible hours, or an attractive financial or benefit package may serve as the selling point.

Interviewing

After advertising, the next step in the process is interviewing. Before or after interviewing, references should be checked carefully and thoroughly. Before interviewing, it is necessary to decide what questions will be asked [5,6]. There are generally two types of interviews, traditional and behavioral [7]. In a traditional interview, questions are asked that have a straightforward answer, for example, "What are your strengths and weaknesses?" or "Describe a typical work week [7]."

In a behavioral interview, questions should be posed to find out if the candidate has the skills necessary for the job. Instead of asking the candidate how they would behave, they are asked how they have behaved in previous experiences. How one behaved in the past generally will indicate how they will behave in the future [7]. A few examples of behavioral interview questions are as follows [7]: "Have you handled a difficult situation with a coworker and, if so, how?" "Tell me about how you worked effectively under pressure." "Can you give an example of a time when you had to deal with a patient who was disgruntled or in uncontrollable pain?"

Questions should be directly related to the job and the job duties the employee will be performing in the position. Certain questions cannot be legally asked of the applicant [5], such as questions related to age, race, color, sex, disability, religion, national origin, pregnancy, and other protected classifications [6].

Pre-employment credentialing

Before an offer is made, the dentist should ask for licenses and credentials to keep on file for legal purposes. It is important for potential candidates to know that maintaining all required credentials is their responsibility. These credentials could include a state license, tuberculosis testing, basic life support training, a handling of biologic hazardous materials certificate, continuing education units, and any other items your practice may require [8].

An offer may be made contingent upon the applicant passing a pre-employment drug screen or national criminal background check. If pre-employment screening will be required, it should be stated in the advertisement. The type of screening may depend on the type of job for which the applicant is being hired. For example, when hiring for the position of billing and collections officer, it would be important to know if an applicant had been previously arrested for embezzlement. The cost of screening varies from state to state [9].

Compensation

As is true for any business, a dental practice is only as strong as the providers and staff it has hired, trained, developed, and retained. People form the foundation and life blood of any organization [10]. A key component to attracting the best, most qualified employees is to establish a competitive compensation package [11]. In traditional terms, compensation is the salary and benefits paid to employees; however, in its broadest sense, compensation may encompass the value of professional development opportunities, training, bonuses and incentives, as well as the provision of services by the dental provider [12].

Salary

In many instances, salary is the single most important factor in determining whether an employee will become a member of the dental practice team.

For this reason, it is critical that the practice owner or trusted office manager keep apprised of salaries being offered in the local and regional market by competing dental practices. In various locations around the country, the demand for qualified dental providers and professionals outpaces the supply; therefore, a practice's ability to first attract and then retain the best talent is becoming more and more critical to its success. To maintain the most recent salary data regarding market salaries, a variety of options exist. One of the simplest options is to call area colleagues and inquire about pay scales. Reviewing the positions posted in the local newspaper may also give you an idea of approximate ranges being offered for certain positions [13]. Yet another, and more technically savvy, approach is to access the vast resources available online. Multiple Web sites exist that will provide salary data based on industry and position description or title. These sites do much of the legwork involved in compiling and even analyzing data to assist in the process of determining appropriate salaries for the dental team.

An additional factor in determining an employee's pay is deciding whether the position is to be paid on an hourly or salaried basis. Among other topics, the Federal Fair Labor Standards Act outlines whether a position can be paid on a salaried basis, also know as exempt [14]. If a position is non-exempt or hourly, the position must be paid at least the minimum wage and be eligible for overtime. Depending on a practice's particular staffing patterns, the use of overtime may create an opportunity to provide additional pay to employees who work longer hours rather than hiring an additional employee.

In certain instances, practice owners may elect to provide compensation to employees based on certain performance goals set by the owner. For example, office staff may receive additional remuneration based on a percentage of payments collected on the date of service or improvements in certain other financial indicators. Similarly, other associates may be paid all or a portion of their salary based on the patients treated, billed charges, dollars collected, or some combination of these factors [15].

The final piece of the salary component involves maintenance and administration of a structure that specifies how and under what criteria an employee may be considered for a salary increase. Procedures for administering increases can range from an "as-needed" basis to a much more formal process of periodic evaluations, typically annually, with increases tied to performance ratings. The types of scoring systems used can vary widely depending on the preferences of the practice owner.

Benefits

In addition to providing a competitive salary to employees, practice owners must also determine the level of benefits offered as part of the overall compensation package. The most common benefits include paid time off for vacation and sick leave, which may be provided individually or grouped together as simply paid time off, commonly known as PTO [16]. There is no federal mandate to provide paid time off, but certain situations are covered under federal regulations with respect to unpaid leave, such as time granted under the Family Medical Leave Act.

As a further means to attract and retain quality employees, practice owners may decide to offer benefit packages that include certain types of insurance. These insurances commonly include health care insurance and life insurance but may be extended to include vision plans, disability plans, and paid professional liability insurance for providers [17]. Although these plans are typically available individually, many state and national professional agencies have developed arrangements with insurers to offer discounted group rates for those belonging to an association, such as a state dental association. The benefit provided to employees can be the ability to access the discounted group rates, or the practice owner may elect as a further benefit to pay all or a portion of selected benefits chosen by the employee.

Additionally, one of the most common benefit options presented to employees is the provision of reduced-fee or no-fee dental services. Although this benefit, if offered, is often capped or otherwise limited, it presents a significant potential allowance for employees.

A further benefit that is becoming more popular is offering some form of retirement plan to employees. There are many options for practice owners, some of which are designed to be more attractive to small business, including employer-sponsored 401(k) plans, Savings Incentive Match Plans for Employees (SIMPLE), and Simplified Employee Pensions (SEPs) [18]. According to the 2000 Small Employer Retirement Survey, among small employers that do sponsor a retirement plan, 47% report that this benefit had a major impact on their ability to hire and retain good employees [18]. Practice owners should consult with tax, accounting, and legal professionals to determine the alternative most suited for a particular practice.

Professional development

Aside from salary and benefits, total compensation packages may include other perquisites such as continuing education or other professional development. These perks may further be segregated into those that are required to obtain or maintain the certification required to perform basic job duties, such as continuing education credit needed for licensure or certification as an expanded duty dental assistant, and those that are strictly for professional development, such as memberships and dues to certain professional organizations. Again, the level of benefit provided can range from allowing for paid time off to attend seminars and conferences to subsidizing the cost of travel, lodging, registration fees, or other expenses associated with attendance at the education or development events. The practice owner may also choose to provide certain training and education opportunities for employees in an effort to impart a better patient experience and to protect the practice from a liability perspective. These training options may include sessions on the Health Insurance Portability and Accountability Act of 1996 (HIPAA), basic life support, sexual harassment, the Occupational Safety and Health Administration (OSHA), and so on. Certain states may also have additional required training courses.

All of the factors alluded to in determining the overall compensation to be offered to a prospective employee or administered for existing employees are best specified in writing to lend clarity. The simplest form of documentation comes in the form of an offer letter. This offer letter may be brief and simply outline compensation proposed and an effective start date. For a more formal and detailed documentation of employment arrangements, such as hiring a provider, the practice owner may elect to require a practice manual or an employment contract. Although several examples of employment contracts are available online, this contract may typically be prepared or reviewed by a legal professional and includes more specific details of working hours, overall compensation, non-compete provisions, and separation of employment, whether resignation or termination. By providing an employment agreement, both the practice owner and the employee have a more defined summary of responsibilities, expectations, and compensation.

Policies and procedures

Every dental practice should seriously consider devising a handbook of policies and procedures for each employee in the practice. These policies should establish, legally define, and document expectations concerning the hours of operation, professional manner, dress code, job tasks, performance evaluations, disciplinary actions, and need for termination if violations occur. These policies and procedures have a significant role in running a successful dental practice.

Hours of operation

Most dentists tend to work more than 32 hours per week while older dentists tend to reduce their hours of operation [19,20]. Some dental practices also offer anticyclic work hours, such as evenings or weekends, or extended work days to accommodate patients who have traditional work hours or who have difficulty taking off work to seek dental treatment. Given these trends, it is essential to identify a flexible work schedule and maintain a work force capable of adapting their operational hours to the needs of the patients and the practice to maintain a competitive and successful edge over the long term.

It is the responsibility of the practice owner to clearly define and display the dental practice's operational hours to patients and the dental team and to give each team member a reasonable amount of time to adjust if circumstances force a change in the operational hours. Because local, state, national, and international labor laws sometimes vary significantly from one another, the practice owner should ensure that the operational hours of the practice location do not violate or conflict with these labor laws and regulations.

Professional conduct

It is also important to establish policies and procedures regarding professional manner and conduct. These policies will significantly define how a dental practice is viewed by the dental team, patients, and other health care professionals. They help affirm responsible and ethical behavior in employees and make it part of their job to get along with colleagues, coworkers, and the patient population [21]. Establishing solid coworker relationships by developing a language of respect and improving communication skills can avoid confrontation, frustration, and misunderstandings. Being caring, courteous, polite, and knowledgeable and communicating these skills to patients help foster patient-dentist, patient-staff, and dentist-staff relationships. These skills develop an atmosphere of comfort and calmness and help reduce tension within the dental team.

In developing a guideline of professional conduct it is advisable to include a policy for smoking or nonsmoking in the work place and to address options for employers and employees dealing with this issue [22,23]. These policies will help decrease friction within the dental team by giving them a clear understanding of the practice's philosophy and how the practice wishes to be perceived by the public. Depending on the country or state or location (ie, public versus private) in which the dental practice operates, laws or regulations might already be in place dictating these policies [24–26].

Dress code

While forming policies for a dental practice, it is important to devise guidelines for work force hygiene and dress code [27]. Work force hygiene and a dress code help the practice, foremost the dentist, establish and improve all aspects of the patient-dentist interaction [28]. Several studies have revealed that appropriate professional attire inspires the patient's trust, confidence, interaction, and perception of the competence of health care professionals [28–30]. Guidelines could be as simple as rules for wearing nametags, jewelry, or cosmetics to more complex rules for wearing street clothes, uniforms, hair styles, and personal hygiene [27]. These guidelines should be clear and descriptive but not discriminatory in nature.

Job descriptions

One of the more stressful parts of managing a dental practice is not necessarily providing care for the patients but dealing with day-to-day staff-related issues [31]. Taking the time to identify, hire, and maintain a resourceful and flexible dental team will likely reduce staff issues and related stress. A key element in this process is developing flexible job descriptions that help employees understand expectations and their potential role in the dental practice. It is imperative that the dental team understand that job descriptions can and will likely evolve in their form as technologic changes and new advances in dentistry occur. Ensuring a flexible job description and a flexible work force will help provide the best possible treatment for patients and maintain a progressive and modern dental practice [32]. Job descriptions also serve as a baseline to improve performance and re-evaluate each staff member's progress [32].

Performance evaluations

Performance evaluations serve as an effective feedback tool for the dental staff and supervisor or evaluator by enforcing strong work ethics and reducing poor conduct in the dental practice [33,34]. They improve the interaction between the dentist and employee and lead to higher incentives and job satisfaction, benefiting the entire dental practice in the short and long term [34].

Performance evaluations should correlate with the job description of the respective employee. Evaluations should be a summary of past performance and a planning session for the future. They should not generate any surprise for the staff member. The performance appraisal serves as legal documentation for promotion, disciplinary action, or termination and should reflect the employee's true performance. The legal implications of inconsistencies cannot be stressed enough as can been seen in the recent media coverage of the firings of eight US attorneys when the reasons for job termination were not consistent with job performance evaluations [35,36].

Research has shown that having multiple competent and knowledgeable people evaluate a person's work performance results in a more accurate appraisal and provides better Equal Employee Opportunity documentation [33]. This process also increases the performance evaluation's perceived fairness [33]. In many dental settings, this multiple rater appraisal system is not possible because the dental team is significantly smaller than in a hospital, university, large multi-site practice group, or corporation. In a small dental practice setting, practice owners must use the more common single rater personnel evaluation system.

The frequency of performance evaluations is another factor to consider when establishing a performance appraisal policy. The practice owner should determine whether they should be performed monthly, quarterly, semi-annually, annually, or every 2 years. Shorter performance evaluation intervals provide quicker constructive and corrective feedback; however, they take away valuable clinical time and do not substitute for corrective advice if needed at the point of occurrence. It is a balancing act that has to be fine tuned and manipulated for each dental practice individually.

Once the performance evaluations are reviewed with the staff member, if corrective action is required, the staff member should be given ample opportunity to actively maneuver their performance to meet or exceed the current standards of the dental practice. When no noticeable improvement occurs or it does not meet the standard of the practice, the dental practice needs to document these developments before considering any disciplinary actions or even termination, because employers do not enjoy the same rights as they once did to fire an employee for a justifiable reason, poor reason, or no reason at all [37,38]. Today, many courtrooms tend to have more sympathy for the employee, making litigation and liability suits against a former employer a credible concern [39].

Dental practice owners can decrease their exposure to employment litigations through vigilant supervision and documentation of the hiring, performance appraisal, and disciplinary process; however, implementing these procedures does not ensure a dental practice legal protection from discharged employees. Moreover, other legal precautions, such as written disclaimers, can head off litigations in employee terminations and discourage plaintiffs' attorneys from pursuing legal action.

Disciplinary and termination policies

When formulating disciplinary policies, the more comprehensive they are, the more protection they might offer an employer from liability following job termination of an employee. These more comprehensive policies could include an oral warning followed by written documentation of the oral warning. If no improvement occurs, the practice owner might want to proceed to one or several written warnings before placing an employee on a probation period which is usually around 90 days. During the probation period, if further disciplinary action is needed, the practice owner may want to place the employee on suspension (ie, unpaid leave for up to 3 days). The final step after suspension is job termination.

A policy for job termination should be included in a policies and procedures handbook for each employee so that they are aware of performance or lack of performance or behavior that will result in termination. Grounds for termination could include, but are not limited to, falsification of the employment records and time records, insubordination, unprofessional conduct which serves to defame or malign the reputation of the dental practice, dishonesty on the job, imperiling the safety of the dental team or the public, possession of a deadly weapon on the dental premise, gambling on the office premises, negligent destruction of dental office property, drug or alcohol abuse while on the job or office premises, fighting, physical assault, physical violence, or the threat of physical violence while on the job, job abandonment, acts which constitute a violation of local, state, national, or international law while on the job or dental practice property, and incarceration in jail following a conviction by a court of law which results in missing at least 5 consecutive working days. Also, it could be the final step after exhausting disciplinary actions.

The disciplinary and termination policy outlined herein should not be considered legal advice and might not be suitable and applicable for every dental practice. It is the responsibility of every practice owner to educate themselves and to possibly seek legal advice before finalizing a disciplinary and termination policy because these policies might conflict with local, state, national, or international laws.

Legal requirements

By law, dental employers must post the Fair Labor Standards Act minimum wage poster in their dental office [40]. Also, OSHA requires the posting of Publication 3165 in all dental offices [41]. The poster outlines the rights of employees and explains the procedure for filing a complaint. These posters must be placed in a conspicuous location where all employees can readily see them. A copy of the OSHA poster may be downloaded or ordered free from OSHA's Web site at www.osha.gov or by calling OSHA's toll free number at 1-800-321-OSHA. A complete list of OSHA regulations for dental offices including those regarding blood borne pathogens, hazards, radiation, exit routes, and electrical safety may be found on their Web site in Title 29 of the Code of Federal Regulations Title 29 (29 CRF). Twenty-four states have adopted their own state occupational safety and health plans [41]. Dentists should contact the OSHA office for more information about regulations specific for their state.

In 1996, HIPPA mandated that all health care providers be assigned a unique identifier, the National Provider Identifier (NPI). Dental offices that employ other dentists should be aware of this regulation and may contact NPI's toll free number at 1-800-465-3203 for more information [42].

OSHA's ionizing radiation standard (29 CFR 1910.1096) mandates that x-ray machines be placed in restricted areas and that employees working in these areas wear radiation monitors. Caution signs may need to be placed in x-ray rooms and on equipment [41]. Individual states also provide laws regarding x-ray safety. Information may be obtained through each state's health and human resources department.

Summary

Technologic changes are leading dentistry into a new era enabling dental practitioners to provide higher quality and more efficient care to their growing patient population, especially an aging baby-boom generation. To accommodate the increase in patient care, existing dental practices are expanding and new dental practices are opening. Most of these practices are faced with similar challenges of identifying, hiring, and retaining a pleasant, competent, and reliable dental team while heading off confrontations within the team.

To build or expand a successful dental practice, the dentist must establish a strong dental team. This process starts with writing a job description for a vacancy that communicates the job expectations, qualifications, and philosophy of the practice. Once the job description is complete, recruitment is initiated by word of mouth or, more formally, by advertising the vacancy in an appropriate publication. After potential candidates are identified, it is always advisable to check their references before interviewing them. The interview offers a good opportunity to see whether the candidate is a suitable match for the dental practice. If a candidate is successful, a job offer should be made contingent on the employee passing a pre-employment credentialing, such as a criminal background check, drug screening test, and verification of job credentials.

Identifying and hiring an excellent candidate is a challenge, but retaining the candidate can become a bigger challenge. It is important to have a competitive compensation package in place. The salary is often the determining compensation criterion for attracting and retaining excellent employees; therefore, the dentist needs to ensure that the salary for a particular job is at market level or even slightly above market level. The market level salary for a particular job can be researched locally or online. Other benefit perks such as vacation, sick leave, professional development, and health and life insurance can also serve as a successful tool for attracting and retaining a strong dental work force.

Even though a competitive salary and benefits package is an important recruitment and retention tool, it does not ensure a successful and smoothly running dental team. Very often, staff-related issues create a stressful working environment. Policies and procedures for each employee should be in place to establish expectations concerning the hours of operation, professional manner, dress code, job tasks, performance evaluations, disciplinary actions, and need for termination if violations occur. Successfully enforcing these policies will reduce conflicts within the dental team, head off litigations, and maintain a successful dental practice in the long term.

Lastly, the dental team must understand and abide by laws and regulations established by government agencies to protect the health and rights of each employee. Most of these laws must be displayed in a conspicuous location within the dental office.

References

[1] Ellis N. Recruiting surgery staff. Br Med J (Clin Res Ed) 1984;289(6436):23–6.

[2] Firth R. Write a job description. Br Med J 1989;298(6683):1306–7.

[3] McNamara C. Employee job descriptions. Adapted from the Field Guide to Leadership and Supervision. 2006. Available at: http://www.manegementhelp.org/staffing/specify/job_desc/job_desc.htm. Accessed March 22, 2007.

[4] Heathfield S. Your guide to human resources. About recruiting stars: top ten ideas for recruiting great candidates. Available at: http://humanresources.about.com/cs/recruiting/a/candidatepool.htm. Accessed March 22, 2007.
[5] Smith L. Interview questions you shouldn't ask. 2007. Available at: http://www.hrhero.com/q&a/061705-questions.shtml. Accessed March 20, 2007.
[6] Doyle A. Illegal interview questions: your guide to job searching. Available at: http://jobsearch.about.com/od/interviewsnetworking/a/illegalinterv.htm. Accessed March 20, 2007.
[7] Doyle A. Behavioral interview: your guide to job searching. Available at: http://jobsearch.about.com/cs/interviews/a/behavioral.htm. Accessed March 20, 2007.
[8] Arturi T. Startups.co.uk build a better business, writing a recruitment advertisement. Available at: http://www.startups.co.uk/Writing_a_recruitment_advertisement.YbhnEAFojdegVw.htm. Accessed March 20, 2007.
[9] University of Kentucky Human Resources Department. Pre-employment National Background Checks (PNBC): frequently asked questions (FAQ). Available at: http://www.uky.edu/HR/HiringOfficials/PDS/BackgroundCheckFAQ.html. Accessed March 27, 2007.
[10] Deal TE, Jenkins WA. Managing the hidden organization. New York: Warner Books; 1994. p. 78.
[11] Heathfield S. Keep your best: retention tips. Available at: http://humanresources.about.com/cs/retention/a/turnover.htm. Accessed July 10, 2007.
[12] Council on Dental Practice. Starting your dental practice: a complete guide. Chicago (IL): American Dental Association; 2001. p. 47–56.
[13] Pelican Applications. Manage your practice human resources. Available at: http://xpractice.com/myp/humanresources.asp. Accessed July 10, 2007.
[14] United States Department of Labor. Handy reference guide to the Fair Labor Standards Act (FLSA). Available at: http://www.dol.gov/esa/regs/compliance/whd/hrg.htm#2. Accessed July 10, 2007.
[15] Levin R. A better practice: employee incentive programs. J Am Dent Assoc 2004;135(5):635–6.
[16] Minnesota Department of Economic Security. What employee benefits can do for you. Available at: http://www.deed.state.mn.us/lmi/__shared/assets/bene4pg11344.pdf. Accessed July 10, 2007.
[17] Key compensation components. Available at: http://www.allbusiness.com/human-resources/compensation/794-1.html. Accessed July 10, 2007.
[18] Devine D, Paladino V. Small firms may be making premature decision not to offer a retirement plan. Available at: http://www.ebri.org/publications/prel/index.cfm?fa=prelDisp&content_id=530. Accessed July 26, 2007.
[19] Waldman HB. NYSDA membership survey: how the components stack up. N Y State Dent J 2000;66(10):20–4.
[20] Walton SM, Byck GR, Cooksey JA, et al. Assessing differences in hours worked between male and female dentists: an analysis of cross-sectional national survey data from 1979 through 1999. J Am Dent Assoc 2004;135(5):637–45.
[21] Sachs Hills L. 25 Tips for getting along with your co-workers. J Med Pract Manage 2006;22(1):26–8.
[22] Ashe RL Jr, Vaughan DH. Smoking in the work place: a management perspective. Employee Relat Law J 1985–1986;11(3):383–406.
[23] Tiede LP, Hennrikus DJ, Cohen BB, et al. Feasibility of promoting smoking cessation in small worksites: an exploratory study. Nicotine Tob Res 2007;9(Suppl 1):83–90.
[24] Siqueira CE, Barbeau E, Youngstrom R, et al. Worksite tobacco control policies and labor-management cooperation and conflict in New York State. New Solut 2003;13(2):153–71.
[25] McCaffrey M, Goodman PG, Kelleher K, et al. Smoking, occupancy and staffing levels in a selection of Dublin pubs pre and post a national smoking ban, lessons for all. Ir J Med Sci 2006;175(2):37–40.

[26] Harteveldt R. The NHS smoking ban takes away people's right to choose. Nurs Times 2006; 102(26):12.
[27] Hills LS. Establishing guidelines for employee dress and hygiene. J Med Pract Manage 2003; 19(1):39–42.
[28] Gooden BR, Smith MJ, Tattersall SJ, et al. Hospitalised patients' views on doctors and white coats. Med J Aust 2001;175(4):219–22.
[29] Rehman SU, Nietert PJ, Cope DW, et al. What to wear today? Effect of doctor's attire on the trust and confidence of patients. Am J Med 2005;118(11):1279–86.
[30] McKinstry B, Wang JX. Putting on the style: what patients think of the way their doctor dresses. Br J Gen Pract 1991;41(348):270, 275–8.
[31] Jupp A. Hiring, staffing policies and productivity. J Am Dent Assoc 2000;131(5):647–50.
[32] Blair DJ. Writing a job description/contract for a dental hygienist in dental practice. J N Z Soc Periodontol 1997;(82):40–5.
[33] Boissoneau RA, Edwards MR. Multiple rater performance appraisals: solutions for hospital personnel. Hosp Health Serv Adm 1985;30(2):54–66.
[34] Singer MG. Performance appraisals: more than just a feedback tool. Legal documentation for employment decisions. Clin Lab Manage Rev 1990;4(4):219–21.
[35] Johnston D, Lipton E. Rove is linked to early query over dismissal. New York: The New York Times; 2007. p. 1.
[36] Cohen A. Editorial observer: why have so many US attorneys been fired? It looks a lot like politics. New York: The New York Times; 2007. p. 20.
[37] Brown F. Limiting your risks in the new Russian roulette–discharging employees. Employee Relat Law J 1982–1983;82(3):380–406.
[38] Elliott CL, Kaiser G. Firing without fear: heading off litigation in employee terminations. Health Prog 1989;70(2):42–5.
[39] Long JE. Limiting liability in employee terminations. Coll Rev 1986;3(1):19–30.
[40] US Department of Labor. Compliance assistance: help navigating DOL laws and regulations. Available at: http://www.dol.gov/osbp/sbrefa/poster/matrix.htm. Accessed July 12, 2007.
[41] US Department of Labor. Occupational Safety and Health Administration. Medical and dental offices: a guide to compliance with OSHA standards. Available at: http://www.osha.gov/Publications/OSHA3187/osha3187.html. Accessed July 12, 2007.
[42] Department of Health and Human Services. National Plan and Provider Enumeration System (NPPES), NPI Registry. Available at: https://nppes.cms.hhs.gov. Accessed July 12, 2007.

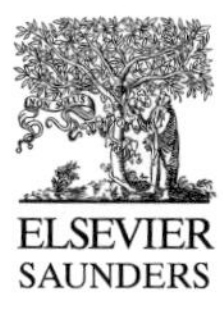
ELSEVIER
SAUNDERS

THE DENTAL CLINICS OF NORTH AMERICA

Dent Clin N Am 52 (2008) 549–562

Insurance Planning for Dentists and Dental Practices

Kenneth C. Thomalla, CPA, CLU, CFPR[a,*], Jeffrey Wherry, CLU, CFPR[b]

[a]*Treloar and Heisel, Inc., 11512 West 183rd Street, Unit NW, Orland Park, IL, USA*
[b]*3132 Wilmington Road, New Castle, PA 16105, USA*

When it comes to overall financial planning, insurance planning is often given little or no attention when, in fact, it is one of the most important parts in the financial planning process. As the old adage goes, a house is only as strong as the foundation it sits upon. The same holds true for your financial livelihood. Insurance planning for the dentist and his or her dental practice should be a top priority for all practitioners.

Hierarchy of financial planning

Proper financial planning follows a defined structure: visualize the future, develop the strategies to accomplish this vision, and then implement the strategies. A dentist would not perform a procedure without first conducting a comprehensive examination and making a diagnosis. Financial strategies, which are among life's most important decisions, must also be made through a coordinated plan based on the same analytic process.

The financial pyramid concept illustrates the hierarchy of financial planning. A proper base forms the foundation to support any strong structure. Financial planning follows the same formula. Start with the base and then move to the next level once the foundational steps are completed. Unfortunately, some dentists skip some elements of the base and move to the next level, ultimately leaving a shaky foundation.

Build your base

The financial base covers five important areas.

* Corresponding author.
E-mail address: kthomalla@th-online.net (K.C. Thomalla).

0011-8532/08/$ - see front matter
doi:10.1016/j.cden.2008.02.007 *dental.theclinics.com*

Emergency fund

All dentists should maintain a strong cash position. Set aside and leave 3 to 6 months' of living expenses in a liquid account, such as a savings account, money market, or other liquid account. This account is not an investment or spending account but rather a fund for emergency expenditures, such as insurance deductibles, transitional expenses to a new practice situation, major home repairs, to cover the waiting period on disability insurance, and other unexpected needs.

Spending plan

Success of a financial plan stems from control of spending and good saving habits. Controlling spending habits and practicing the discipline of delayed gratification are often difficult financial tasks for a dentist. All practitioners should prepare a budget with a fixed spending limit. Spending can be adjusted upward as income increases. Consistency helps to ensure the discipline of a spending plan; thus, a predetermined monthly draw should be established to cover fixed spending.

Often, it helps to create a cash flow map—a predetermined distribution of your monthly and periodic income. For instance, a certain amount of dollars might be directed each month to:

- Monthly checking for spending purposes
- A tax account
- A college savings account
- A periodic spending account for vacations and other recurring expenses

Quarterly and annual distributions might be earmarked for retirement and other accumulation accounts.

Follow wise debt rules

Generally, personal debt, not including practice acquisition loans, should not exceed 30% of gross income. This may be unrealistic in the first year of practice but should be adhered to in following years. Additional debt rules to observe include the following:

- Recognize the difference between "good debt" and "bad debt." Good debt buys an appreciating asset, such as your home, or an income stream, such as your practice income. Good debt includes student loans, practice loans, and home mortgages. Bad debt purchases include depreciating assets or expenditures with no residual value, often at high interest rates. Credit card debt and consumer debt are examples of bad debt.
- Do not accelerate debt payment if the interest rate on the loan is less than the rate of return of a moderate growth investment.

Create a basic estate plan

Most new practitioners do not think much about estate planning; in fact, most new practitioners do not even realize that they have an estate. Considering that many finish dental school or residency with loans in excess of $200,000, it is easy to see why many believe they do not have to plan for their estate distribution.

Many of these individuals actually have items that they would like to pass to an intended recipient, however. Thus, no matter the net worth of an individual, a will is often the minimum estate planning strategy needed by all. Later in life, and beyond the scope here, there are other estate planning tools necessary to ensure that an estate is distributed in the intended and most tax-efficient manner.

When an individual dies without a will, it is known as dying intestate. If a person dies intestate, his or her estate is distributed by the laws of the state in which he or she resides. Often, the distribution rules established by the states are not in sync with how a decedent would like to have his or her estate distributed. For example, most new practitioners would like to have their spouses receive their entire estate on their death. Some intestate laws distribute these funds to the spouse and to children and other family members, however. Additionally, a will provides a vehicle for parents to determine who takes care of their children on their death. Without a will, the courts determine who the guardian is for minor children.

Furthermore, in the absence of a will, the state determines the executor, and it may not be the person the doctor desires. Initiating a will allows the doctor to choose the executor, saving his or her survivors significant legal footwork at an already difficult time.

Purchase insurance

Insurance is another important pillar of your financial base.

Everybody faces certain perils in life that can result in a significant financial loss. Examples of these perils are premature death, disability, catastrophic medical expenditures, property damage or theft, and professional and personal litigation.

The purchase of insurance transfers the risk to the insurance company, providing money when none exists to replace the loss from these perils. Insurance trades a potentially unaffordable loss, the cost of the peril, for a known affordable cost, the premium. Typically, only unaffordable losses should be insured, even if the risk for occurrence is relatively low. The remainder of this article discusses personal and business insurance plans that are required by most dentists.

Personal insurance

Disability income insurance

A dentist's ability to perform his or her occupation is, in effect, the "production line." Inability to perform these functions because of a disability can cause great financial loss. Disability income insurance should be purchased by a new practitioner immediately on entering practice, if not while a dental student.

Disability income insurance is purchased in monthly increments. Companies limit the amount of available coverage to approximately 40% to 60% of income. The amount of coverage available, as a proportion of income, decreases as income increases. Income documentation must be provided to purchase benefits, although dental students and residents often may buy a stated amount of coverage without proof of income.

Several important provisions must be evaluated when purchasing disability income insurance:

- Policy ownership: a "noncancelable and guaranteed renewable" policy prohibits the insurance company from increasing rates or changing policy provisions to the detriment of the policyholder. It is the recommended type of policy for dental professionals and is typically available through local agents. Many association group policies are "conditionally renewable," which allows the insurance company to increase rates and alter policy definitions. Although conditionally renewable plans often have lower rates than noncancelable and guaranteed renewable policies, a rate or definition change could leave the dentist with inadequate coverage. Some professional associations endorse noncancelable and guaranteed renewable policies with a discounted premium. These plans often offer the best of both worlds—strong definitions at more affordable rates.
- Definition of total disability: the best policies pay benefits when you are unable to perform the "material and substantial duties of your regular occupation." A true own occupation definition pays full benefits if you cannot perform your occupation even if you go to work in another occupation. Rates for true own occupation policies are typically the most expensive. A modified version of own occupation is one in which benefits are paid if you cannot perform your regular occupation as long as you choose not to work at another occupation. Under these policies, income loss benefits may actually be paid under a partial disability rider while engaged in another occupation.
- Partial or residual disability: in many cases, a dentist may have an illness or injury yet still work part-time at his or her occupation. Partial disability, often referred to as "residual disability," pays partial benefits based on income loss when the dentist is disabled but still working at his or her regular occupation. Some companies include residual disability in the base contract, although others provide it as an optional rider.

- Elimination period: benefits usually do not begin on the first day of disability. An elimination period, typically 90 days from the first day of disability, must be satisfied, after which benefits commence.
- Benefit period: the length of time benefits are paid during a disability is referred to as the "benefit period." Choose a benefit period that pays benefits to the age of 65 years, at a minimum. Benefit payments for life, depending on age at the onset of the disability, are available as an optional rider on some plans, although others might offer a rider that makes contributions to retirement plans during a disability.
- Cost-of-living rider: even at a modest 3% inflation rate, income has to double over 24 years to keep pace with inflation. If a disability were to occur at a young age, benefits must increase to maintain purchasing power. An important optional rider, cost-of-living (COLA), increases benefits during a disability and is usually tied to changes in the consumer price index (or set as a fixed rate).
- Additional purchase option or future increase option: to buy disability insurance, a prospective insured must prove good health. Under a noncancelable guaranteed renewable policy, the insurance company cannot later restrict or cancel the policy based on negative changes in the insured's health. The insurance company can refuse to increase coverage, or increase at less than favorable terms, if the insured has subsequent health problems, however. Most companies offer optional riders that allow the dentist to purchase additional coverage later, as long as his or her income meets stated benefit issue limits, with the same terms and conditions of the existing policy, even if the insured were to experience a health problem that would otherwise render him or her uninsurable.

Life insurance

A dentist may need life insurance for three specific situations:

- Personal needs: to provide income for family members.
- Collateral for a business loan: many banks require life insurance to be assigned as collateral for practice loans.
- Funding for a business buyout agreement: life insurance provides funding to purchase remaining practice value from a deceased partner's estate.

How much coverage is appropriate? In the case of loan collateral or buyout agreements, the amount of coverage is equal to the stated need of the loan or agreement. Programming coverage for personal needs is more nuanced, however. Often, stated guidelines, such as "eight times income," may overinflate or underinflate the actual need. A basic mathematic computation as stated here provides a more accurate figure:

1. Lump sum needs: amount needed to pay off debt and prefund other obligations.

2. Income needs: determine the present value of the annual income required by the family and for how long.
3. Add lump sum needs and income needs, and subtract existing liquid assets.

This formula does not factor in potential social security benefits or inflation. A qualified insurance professional may use computation software for more advanced calculations.

Term and permanent are the two general classifications of life insurance that are available.

Term life

Term life insurance covers temporary needs, providing only pure protection without any cash accumulation. Rates start low but increase, becoming prohibitively expensive at some point in time. Multiple term life policies are available, including term with annually increasing premiums and level premium terms of 10, 15, 20, and 30 years. With level-rate plans, premiums increase exponentially at the end of the stated period. A buyer should purchase the term policy with a level premium period that corresponds to how long coverage is required.

Permanent life

Permanent life insurance provides policy protection for life and cash accumulation within the policy. Premiums are set for the term of the contract while the policy develops an accumulation value on a tax-deferred basis. At some point in time, the policy cash value may be sufficient to reduce or eliminate the premium or be drawn on as income. Permanent life insurance is sold in several variations, including whole life, universal life, and variable life. Although significantly higher in premium than term life at the outset, permanent life costs less over a lifetime.

Because of the low cost, term life is likely to provide the bulk of coverage throughout most of a dentist's career. Permanent life may also be implemented to augment retirement and estate planning strategies and to provide financial flexibility later in life.

Long-term care insurance

Over the years, long-term care insurance (LTCI) has become part of a financial plan for new and seasoned practitioners. It was always common practice to put off the purchase of LTCI until the age of 60 years or older. Most of these individuals purchased coverage only after dealing with long-term care services provided to a parent. As the statistics are starting to show, however, many young people use long-term care services. As a result, the age of issue for LTCI is beginning to drop. For the younger practitioner, LTCI is purchased along with medical and disability insurance to protect against the catastrophic event that requires long-term care services.

The older dental practitioner may purchase LCTI as an estate preservation tool. As one plans and saves for retirement, in addition to poor investment decisions and overspending, the need for long-term care services can deplete an estate fairly quick.

LCTI is structured similar to disability insurance. The purchaser has some flexibility in choosing the options best suited for his or her situation. Daily benefit, elimination period, and benefit period are the first items to consider when purchasing LTCI. The daily benefit amount should be matched closely to one's surrounding community in which care may be provided. With the addition of a cost-of-living rider, the benefit amount should increase as the insured ages. Hopefully, this can help to keep the policy in line with increasing long-term care costs. The elimination period dictates the time frame as to when benefits begin, although many companies offer benefit periods of 3, 5, 10, and an unlimited number of years.

Rates for LCTI are not normally guaranteed, although some insurance companies offer limited year payment options guaranteeing that no further premium payments are due after the stated number of years.

Auto insurance

Although most states require the purchase of auto liability insurance, individuals still need to be aware of the risk involved with being underinsured. Most individuals insure their autos with the following coverage: liability, comprehensive, collision, and uninsured or underinsured motorists. Liability coverage insures a driver against claims made by other drivers as a result of an accident. Bodily injury, property damage, and medical payments are the three components of liability protection.

Many states mandate certain limits of liability coverage and, especially if a dental professional has a personal umbrella policy, his or her limits far exceed those required by his or her state. Those without a personal umbrella liability policy need to ensure that their auto liability coverage is adequate. A dentist exposed to an auto liability claim risks his or her personal assets if underinsured.

Comprehensive and collision protection insures the physical damage to the insured's automobile. Comprehensive coverage insures the damage arising by a covered peril other than collision. Uninsured or underinsured coverage protects the dentist in case the other driver who was responsible for an accident lacks adequate coverage of his or her own. In this case, the dentist's coverage essentially takes the place of the driver who did not have adequate auto insurance.

Because many new automobiles provide roadside assistance or similar protection, it may not be necessary to carry towing and rental coverage on an auto insurance policy.

Home owners' or rental insurance

Before discussing the different types of property coverage, it is imperative to begin with a discussion regarding the differences between property and casualty policies (PC) and life and health policies (LH). The average consumer often thinks that as long as the premiums are paid, the policy owner is entitled to the benefits under a policy. This assumption is true in that an insurance company pays a covered claim as long as the premiums are paid. The amount to be paid depends on the concept of insurable interest, however. For a PC policy, you must have an insurable interest at the time of the claim. This means that if one's property coverage is listed on the policy at $200,000, although the property is only worth $150,000 at the time of the claim, the insured would only recover $150,000. This is in contrast to an LH policy, such as term life insurance. If the insured dies and the policy was underwritten and issued for $200,000, at the death of the insured, the beneficiary would receive $200,000 under a covered claim. This concept is important, especially when considering the number of properties that may be owned by a dental practitioner.

Home owners' coverage is PC insurance for a true single family home, a condo that one owns, or a home or apartment that is rented by the dentist. Home owners' coverage for a single family home provides protection for the entire home and structures located on the property. The most significant difference with a condo policy is that the condo policy pays benefits for the "drywall in." A master policy, purchased by the condo association, usually covers the exterior of the building. A condo owner must review the association coverage to ensure that the two policies mesh. Overlapping coverage may cost a little more; however, having a gap in coverage can be disastrous. Renter's coverage usually just covers the personal property owned by the renter. The building owner should have a policy covering the real property of the premises.

The insurance limits on any of these policies can be written on a guaranteed replacement basis or replacement basis. Guaranteed replacement means that the insurance company pays a covered claim regardless of the limit on the policy. Obviously, if the loss is lower than the limit, the insured receives the lesser of the two because of the concept of insurable interest. If the loss is greater than the insured limit, however, the policy holder is in a great position and would receive the larger amount. There are many times when an insured may intentionally underinsure to save premium dollars knowing that full coverage is provided under this clause. Many insurance companies have eliminated the guaranteed replacement clause because of this situation.

Replacement value means that as long as the policy limit is equal to at least 80% of the actual home's replacement cost, the loss is paid up to the policy limit. This clause is reasonable and ensures that policy owners take responsibility to insure property for its fair value. Additionally, by not requiring that 100% of the value be insured, this allows for some buffer room if reconstruction costs increase and the policy owner is not timely with increasing his limits. An inflation rider added to the policy helps to keep policy limits escalating as building costs increase.

A typical home owners' policy has additional coverage for general liability and several secondary limits. One such limit is for such items as jewelry, artwork, and musical instruments. These limits are usually relatively low; therefore, many items need to be "scheduled." When an item is scheduled, the entire appraised value is insured and coverage is usually broadened. For example, most policies limit jewelry coverage to $2500 for theft or loss attributable to a covered claim. A $10,000 diamond ring can be scheduled, and therefore insured for $10,000. Additionally, it may even be possible to recover the entire costs if the ring is lost, which is not a loss normally covered under the base policy. All valuable pieces of personal property should be scheduled to maintain appropriate coverage on the item.

Medical insurance

Purchasing medical insurance is may be one of the toughest financial decisions in the dental office, because the dentist must determine if this is going to be an employee benefit deductible through the office. Many factors come into this decision, including the health of the dentist(s), ability to attract qualified staff, and the dentist's own moral compass. If the dentist chooses not to provide medical insurance to the staff, he might still be able to purchase outside of the practice and deduct the costs depending on his business structure.

There are primarily four types of medical insurance: health maintenance organization (HMO), preferred provider organization (PPO), traditional, and health savings account (HSA). HMOs require the insured to stay within the network. These types of plans normally require that the insured visit his primary care provider, or gatekeeper, before visiting a specialist. A PPO eliminates the gatekeeper, allowing for greater flexibility as compared with an HMO. Traditionally, a PPO stresses preventive care and provides for annual check-ups. Traditional medical coverage provides for benefits after an annual deductible is met by the insured. With traditional medical coverage, after the deductible, usual and customary expenses are fully covered subject to the policy's copayment clause.

An HSA is one of the new consumer-driven medical plans. Essentially, it allows the dentist or his employees to deposit money, before taxes, into an account while increasing the deductible under the medical insurance policy.

Medical expenses, up to the deductible, can be paid from the deposit account, or the deposit account can be left to grow over the years, tax deferred. HSAs are better suited for the healthier dentist who will not exhaust the HSA deposit account each year.

Personal umbrella liability insurance

Because of the increased lawsuit risk, all dental professionals should consider a personal umbrella liability insurance policy. An umbrella policy sits on top of other coverage, such as auto and homeowners. The umbrella policy provides an additional layer of liability protection over these base policies. Thus, if an auto policy has a $500,000 liability limit and the umbrella policy has a limit of $2,000,000, the insured has a potential limit of $2,500,000 against a covered liability claim attributable to an auto accident. The term *umbrella* is used because the one umbrella limit covers all the underlying base policies. The limit of umbrella coverage is an individual consideration based on net worth and other risk factors.

Business insurance

Professional liability (malpractice) insurance

Professional liability, or malpractice insurance, is the backbone of any asset protection plan for a dental professional. Over the few years, professional liability premium rates have stabilized. The general dentist typically has premiums rates that are lower than those of most physicians.

The two most common types of professional liability coverage are occurrence and claims-made. Occurrence type coverage provides for a new limit each year of practice. Essentially, one is insured for the procedure performed in a given year, regardless of when a claim may be filed. Thus, if a dental professional practices 30 years, an occurrence policy provides for 30 separate layers of coverage, 1 for each year of practice. This abundance of coverage would help to protect the dentists in the case of claims attributable to procedures taking place over multiple years.

Claims-made coverage was introduced as a way to lower initial premiums for the insured while limiting liability to the insurance company. Claims-made coverage provides insurance protection when a malpractice claim is made against a practitioner, regardless of when the procedure occurred. Unlike occurrence coverage, a limit for claims-made coverage moves with the insured. Throughout a 30-year practice, a dental professional with claims-made coverage has one limit in a given year that must provide coverage for claims attributable to all current and prior years of practice.

Claims-made coverage is initially less expensive when compared with occurrence coverage; however, over a practitioner's career, the premium difference is relatively minor, because the premiums for a claims-made policy increase each of the first 5 years.

Professional liability limits vary between companies but usually start at $1 million to $3 million. The first number indicates a maximum limit for a given year per claim, whereas the second number is the total limit for all claims in a given year. Some believe that dentists should purchase as much professional liability insurance as they can, whereas others look at the scope of their practice to determine the adequate amount of coverage. In either case, it is important to remember that a claim against an insured can extend past insurance to the practice and personal assets of the dentist.

A consent clause under professional liability insurance dictates when an insurance company can settle a claim. Pure consent means that the insured has the final approval as to when and if a claim is settled versus litigating until the end. This is the best definition available and gives the dentist ultimate control over his claim. Many companies offer an arbitration clause. Under this clause, three or more people evaluate the merits of the claim to determine if it should be settled or litigated. The last type of consent is a silent consent clause. Sometimes referred to as a "hammer clause," consent of this type is held only by the insurance company. The dentist really has no say in the settlement of a claim under a silent consent clause.

Office overhead insurance

Personal disability insurance pays benefits for the loss of personal income attributable to an injury or sickness. Office overhead insurance coverage insures the fixed overhead of a dental office. Examples of some of the covered fixed expenses include rent, staff salaries, utilities, telephone, professional fees, and employment taxes. Office overhead coverage is needed by individual and group practices.

Although personal disability insurance and office overhead coverage are quite similar, some differences should be discussed. First, the elimination period for an office overhead policy should be shorter than that of a disability policy. Most planners recommend a 30-day elimination period to ensure that the fixed office expenses are covered without needing to use business or personal savings. Second, the benefit period for an office overhead policy should match the need. Because office overhead coverage is a reimbursement type policy, expenses are only reimbursed if the expenses are the responsibility of the disabled dentist. Thus, if a buy-sell agreement calls for the disabled partner to sell his shares after 12 months of a disability, it would not benefit him to have a 24-month benefit period on his office overhead plan. The additional 12 months of benefits, after the sale, would never be realized by the disabled practitioner.

Taxation of benefits is another difference between office overhead and personal disability insurance. Office overhead insurance benefits are generally nontaxable to the practice even though the premiums are deductible by the practice. This is in contrast to a personal disability plan. If a practice is structured under a regular "C" corporation and elects to set up a qualified sick pay plan, personal disability premiums can be deducted as a business expense. Deducting personal disability premiums causes benefits paid under this policy to become taxable, however. Therefore, it is usually not recommended to pay personal disability premiums with pretax dollars because of the significant taxable event at the time of a claim.

The option to increase an office overhead policy is similar to those contained within a personal disability policy and should always be added to the base coverage. This option allows increases without completing any additional medical underwriting and provides for increased flexibility in future years.

Business owner's policy, workers' compensation, employment practices liability insurance

A business owner's policy (BOP) is a PC type policy that contains numerous benefits. It is important to know what is covered under a BOP in relation to the contents coverage. Such items as equipment, furnishings, and other personal business property are easily determinable as contents. The insured value of real property, or property that is affixed to the space, is not always easily determined because of the previously discussed concept of insurable interest. Thus, a BOP only insures expenses for which an insurable interest exists at the time of a claim. Many times, an office lease is not clear or the practitioner does not understand who is responsible for the build-out of the dental office. Although it is sometimes the responsibility of the landlord, more often, the build-out is the responsibility of the tenant (practice). Therefore, a lease must be written clearly and reviewed by the landlord and the dental practice to ensure that both parties clearly understand who is responsible for the office build-out and that their respective BOP policy contains the required content limit to provide adequate protection against loss.

Many dentists own the building in which their practice is located; thus, it is important to keep an "at-arms-length" lease between the parties. Having a contractually clear and strong lease may help to avoid complications at claim time.

In addition to the content coverage, a BOP has a wide array of other coverage to protect the dentist against loss. General liability, dental waste disposal, employee theft, and accounts receivable are a few examples of the additional coverage found in a BOP.

Workers' compensation coverage protects the dental practice against claims arising out of employment-related sickness and injury. Most states mandate workers' compensation that covers medical and disability payments for an employee. An owner/officer of a practice usually has a choice whether to be covered under the office's workers' compensation policy. It is imperative that if one decides to opt out of workers' compensation coverage, he or she is sure that his or her medical insurance does not exclude claims covered under workers' compensation law. A significant gap in coverage could occur if the practitioner is not covered under his or her medical and workers' compensation insurance.

Because the risk for employment-related lawsuits continues be a risk to all practices, employment practices liability insurance (EPLI) may help to lessen the concern. An EPLI policy guards an employer against employment lawsuits related to hiring, firing, and sexual harassment claims. Coverage can be in the form of defense cost or indemnity payments. Occasionally, this coverage can be purchased as a rider to a BOP; however, higher limits may not be available as a rider. A stand-alone EPLI policy provides for higher limits and the richest contractual features.

Disability and life insurance buyout insurance

Any association of two or more dentists should have an agreement to transfer shares of a practice on the death or disability of one of the partners or shareholders. Regardless of the practice structure (C-corporation, S-corporation, limited liability corporation [LLC], limited liability practice [LLP], or other), most buyout agreements are structured as a cross-purchase or entity purchase.

A cross-purchase buyout agreement states that if one partner becomes disabled or dies, the other partner(s) has first right to buy his or her share of the practice. Under a cross-purchase agreement, it is assumed that the entity is not involved in the sale transaction.

There are tax benefits related to alternative minimum tax (AMT) and subsequent sales related to a cross-purchase. In practices with more than two owners, however, a cross-purchase agreement may be cumbersome when funding with insurance because of the multiple insurance policies needed to insure all the partners.

Under an entity buyout agreement, the entity itself buys the shares from a disabled dental partner or his estate. Essentially, the shares are redeemed, and retired, by the practice, and the other partners' percentage of ownership increases because of the reduction of total outstanding shares. An entity buyout agreement is beneficial when there are more than two partners in a practice. If insurance is purchased to fund an entity buyout agreement, the practice is the owner and beneficiary of each of the policies insuring the partners. A buyout agreement usually contains a clause for death and disability.

The death provision is best funded with term life insurance. The length of the term guarantee should coincide with the length of time the respective partner plans on practicing. For example, a 30-year-old dentist who plans on practicing for an additional 30 years should purchase a 30-year level-term plan.

Many practices choose not to fund the disability portion of a buyout agreement. Some practices believe that if a partner becomes disabled, a newly hired associate should pay off the disabled partner. This may seem logical in some areas, but care needs to be taken because of the lack of certainty of a practice finding a suitable replacement dentist. A disability buyout insurance policy helps to fund the disability provision and to provide peace of mind, for all the partners, that the disabled partner receives the agreed-on price at the time of the buyout. The going concern risk is eliminated when a buyout agreement is funded with life and disability insurance.

There are a myriad of insurance products available for the dentist and his dental practice. Care must be taken to ensure that all risks have been reviewed and the appropriate risks covered with an insurance plan. Taking the time to solidify your base helps to ensure a strong financial plan for years to come.

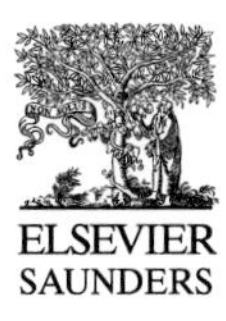

ELSEVIER
SAUNDERS

THE DENTAL CLINICS OF NORTH AMERICA

Dent Clin N Am 52 (2008) 563–577

Risk Management Techniques for the General Dentist and Specialist

Harry Dym, DDS[a,b,c,*]

[a]*Department of Dentistry and Oral Maxillofacial Surgery, The Brooklyn Hospital Center, 121 Dekalb Avenue, Brooklyn, NY 11201, USA*
[b]*Woodhull Hospital, Brooklyn, NY, USA*
[c]*Department of Oral and Maxillofacial Surgery, Columbia University College of Dental Medicine, New York, NY, USA*

Medical malpractice has been with us for hundreds of years, with the first recorded case in the United States occurring in 1794 in the state of Connecticut [1]. All malpractice claims are based on the allegation that the plaintiff was owed some duty by the doctor and that duty was breached, resulting in injury. To obtain a judgment of negligence by the treating doctor, the plaintiff must prove four elements:

Pre-existing duty
Breach of duty
Damage
Causal link

Doctors are not obligated or legally required to treat all patients, but once treatment has passed the consultation phase, the courts usually consider that a doctor–patient relationship has been established. The care provided must be appropriate, according to the community "standard of care," and the plaintiff must then establish that a "breach" of duty has occurred by getting "experts" to offer testimony that the standard of care was not met.

The plaintiff must also establish that damages resulted from the defendant's actions and show a "proximate" cause (ie, no other events occurred that could have caused the damage to happen) linking the treatment to the damages sustained.

* Department of Dentistry and Oral Maxillofacial Surgery, The Brooklyn Hospital Center, 121 Dekalb Avenue, Brooklyn, NY 11201.

E-mail address: hdymdds@yahoo.com

0011-8532/08/$ - see front matter
doi:10.1016/j.cden.2008.02.011

Anatomy of a malpractice claim

Because malpractice litigation is something doctors do not think about routinely, it is important to be knowledgeable about the legal process and practice of malpractice claims.

Most states allow a period of 3 years from the time the patient knew about the injury for a malpractice claim to go forward (referred to as the statute of limitations); this period is extended to 3 years beyond the age of majority for minors. The first notice of a possible malpractice situation will be a document received by the dentist from the plaintiff's counsel requesting records of treatments, which must be accompanied by a release for medical/dental information, signed by the patient. The doctor is obligated to send copies (never originals) of all requested chart materials: radiographs, models, progress notes, patient history, and operating reports. Records must be released even if the patient has not paid any outstanding office form–related fees. The doctor should never engage the plaintiff's counsel in conversation about the patient or the case in question. The doctor's malpractice insurance carrier must be informed in a timely fashion of any request for patient records that may involve a potential malpractice claim.

This request is often followed by the doctor being served with a "summons and complaint," which is often a document filled with exaggeration and significant hyperbole meant to raise doubts and pangs of guilt in the defendant. The doctor should not doubt him/herself or become overly emotional by this summons document (these feelings are, after all, the effect the plaintiff's counsel wishes to elicit) but rather, he/she should go about the business of helping to assemble a good defense with his/her counsel.

Following the summons and complaint, the doctor will begin to have conversations with his/her defense counsel, which are privileged and not subject to disclosure with the plaintiff. It is advisable to sequester the patient's records at this time for safe keeping.

Once litigation has begun, the process of "discovery" ensues. Discovery consists of interrogatories (a series of written questions presented to each side) followed by sworn oral testimony (depositions) by the patient and the doctor. Experts for both sides will evaluate the records and the appropriateness of care delivered to help flush out issues and prepare for trial.

Not all claims wind up in court; some never going forward after the "discovery" phase and others are settled, possibly to avoid open court trials.

Alternatives to litigation

Most states have a "peer review" process sponsored by the state dental society to help resolve disputes between patients and dentists regarding quality-of-care issues and appropriateness of treatment. This procedure is a formal process in which both parties sign an agreement to submit to a review, and in some states, the parties also agree to waive their rights to sue each other for payment or malpractice. In most states, the findings of the peer review committee are privileged and not discoverable should a trial follow, and any payment made by the doctor to the patient is not reported to the national data bank.

Mediation is another form of dispute resolution. A mediator hears opening statements from both involved parties and then hears separate testimony from each. The mediator then attempts to move both parties independently toward an acceptable middle ground for a negotiated settlement.

Arbitration is still another method of dispute resolution. The procedure is similar to a trial, with the arbitrator acting as judge and jury. The parties may accept the decision and settle or move on to a full trial.

Risk-reduction strategies

Malpractice claims focus on three areas of practice: poor communication/rapport, lack of informed consent, and faulty record keeping [2].

Many dentists/physicians think of excellence in terms of technical expertise and successful outcomes because that is the frame of reference first begun in dental/medical school and carried on into residency training. Patients, however, will often gauge quality of care using other guideposts. They will view quality of care as it relates to

- Staff performance and attitude
- Doctor's affability, attitude, and willingness to listen to, and consider, all questions
- Cleanliness of the office
- Level of communication
- Accessibility

It is the patient's perception of the quality of care received that will often tip the scale in favor of the doctors, so careful attention to staff and office policies is vital to maintaining an overall strategy of risk reduction. As part of this strategy, one should not forget to maintain medical/dental equipment in good operational condition and to keep all necessary inventories up to date. Quality radiographs (plain or digital) are vital to good record keeping, along with having all equipment in good operational order.

Informed consent

A landmark 1914 court case (Schloendorff v Society of New York Hospitals) [3] helped define the laws of informed patient consent. "Every human being of adult years and sound mind has a right to determine what shall be done with his/her own body... and a surgeon who operates without the patient's consent commits an assault for which he/she is liable in damages."

Clearly, the court has ruled that consent before surgery must be obtained, but the courts are silent as to how the consent must be obtained and documented. During the years since, risk managers have developed the following recommendations regarding the informed consent process:

1. The taking of consent is not merely a signature on a preprinted form but is really an on-going process that may include (a) verbal discussion, (b) educational materials (videos, CD-ROMs, pamphlets), (c) consent videos, and (d) documentation of the process in the patient's record.
2. The consent discussion should not be delegated to staff personnel; it should be done by the doctor him/herself.

The doctor–patient discussion is the most critical part of the informed consent process, not the signed consent form.

Ideally, the informed consent process should be a written document specific to the procedure being performed because verbal consents are soon forgotten by the patient. The informed consent is composed of several key elements (Box 1).

Communications

Hycke and Hycke [4] interviewed 500 patients who had contacted law firms regarding personal injury lawsuits and found that 55% listed a poor relationship with their doctor as the precipitating factor in their reason to seek legal representation. Clearly, the treating doctor and staff must strive to establish a good rapport (in a short time) with their patient, because this rapport will play a critical role in the ongoing relationship.

Many patients are anxious about visiting the dentist and are often angry and resentful. The doctor and staff must realize this and work diligently to gain their trust (Boxes 2 and 3).

A communication breakdown may occur in the following situations:

Practitioner does not return telephone call.
Practitioner does not answer questions.
Practitioner is too busy to talk and listen.
Practitioner does not explain.
Staff members are not attentive listeners.
Staff members did not explain what they were going to do.

Documentation

Complete patient records are not only vital to good patient care but a legal requirement by most state dental boards. Failure to maintain such records could lead to a loss of license to practice. A complete dental record

- Complies with licensure and accreditation standards
- Facilitates diagnosis and treatment of the patient
- Serves as basis for defense of potential malpractice claim
- Provides basis for communication with different health care members.

Box 1. Key elements of informed consent

Consent should always be obtained by the treating doctor, ideally at a separate consultation visit; it should only be obtained at the time of care if an emergent surgical procedure is required.

Additional educational materials, videos, textbooks, and picture brochures should be used, if available, to help educate the patient about the prepared treatment plan.

When the patient does not understand English, a translator must be present and that fact documented in the patient's chart.

Consent for minors (under age 18 in most states) must be obtained by a parent or legal guardian; however, if urgent care is needed, telephone consent is often acceptable if the parent cannot leave work or is out of town. Patients who are under 18 and are married or have children are able to give consent.

If the patient refuses treatment that the doctor believes is vitally important to his/her future health, this fact should be documented in the patient's chart; many doctors use a special "refusal care" form.

The patient should be advised of the risks of the proposed treatment and the risks of no treatment.

The patient should be advised of alternatives to the proposed treatment.

The patient should be advised of the cost of treatment.

No guarantees of results or outcomes should be made.

Consent should be discussed at separate time from the planned surgical procedure; the patient should be allowed to take the consent form home, which allows time to think about the procedure.

Informed consent forms for surgical procedures performed by oral and maxillofacial surgeons are the standard of care, though this is not the national standard among general dentists and other dental specialists.

- Provides quality assurance data
- Serves as the means to obtain proper reimbursement and helps substantiate billing codes

The ideal chart size is 8.5 × 11 inches, not the small card system that offers little room for information and is always difficult to read. Each patient should have a separate record with all supplementary documents (radiographs, path reports, and so forth) contained in one file. Entries must be made in a timely manner and never altered in response to a subpoena.

Box 2. Improving interactions with patients during examinations/consultations

Once the examination or consultation begins, the dentist should keep in mind these suggestions for more successful communications:

- Greet the patient by name and use the patient's name during the conversation.
- Sit down so that you are at eye level with the patient, and maintain eye contact.
- Scan the problem list for what you perceive as the most important problem, and let the patient know that you will address that one first because you want to make sure it is discussed before you run out of time.
- In pursuing a line of questioning to establish a diagnosis, launching questions without any "lead-in" can feel like an interrogation for some patients. Instead, try prefacing your questions with a reassuring statement that shows concern for the patient and conveys that your purpose in asking some questions is to determine what is wrong and how you might remedy it.
- You may need to ask the patient to make another appointment if time does not allow an evaluation of all the problems on the patient's list, which indicates that, even though all problems may not be addressed at this visit, they will not be dismissed.
- Once the patient begins to discuss his/her problems, practice listening for at least 2 or 3 minutes before you say anything. Show that you are listening by leaning forward and reacting to the patient's body language.
- If you need to turn away from a patient who is in the chair or you have to leave the room, explain where you are going and when you will return. Do not just leave the room.
- Try to become acquainted with the patient on a personal level, asking questions about the patient's work or hobbies during the initial visit. Keep a sheet with this information on the inside cover of the chart or in another easily accessible section and glance at it before meeting with the patient. Discussing personal details while addressing the patient's problems indicates your interest in the whole person.
- Again, facilitate patient interaction and information exchange by using probing, open-ended questions, such as, "What do you think caused this problem to happen?"

Box 3. Tips for managing the difficult patient

The following tips can help improve interactions with difficult patients:

- Be consistent (especially important in a team-driven clinic environment).
- Be persistent.
- Be adaptable.
- Be calm, so the patient mirrors calm behavior.
- Accept the humanness of the patient/family.
- Demonstrate courteous behavior.
- Establish a trusting relationship.
- Show patience.
- Show caring.
- Be attentive.
- Be nonjudgmental.
- Treat the patient as you would want yourself or your loved ones to be treated.
- Show physical and psychologic comfort to the patient.
- Maintain follow-up; do not lose track of patient's care.

In the face of difficult behavior, be sure to respond promptly to concerns, knowledge deficits, and misunderstandings by using the following techniques:

- Intervene.
- Identify the sources of the patient's concern or anxiety.
- Respond to the patient's concern or concerns.
- Try to understand the patient's point of view.
- Share perceptions with the patient about his/her behavior and how the behavior affects the patient and others.

Entries are best made by the doctor because staff entries expose the doctor to a weakened defense if the case should lead to litigation.

Each patient visit should be recorded with the date and a clear, comprehensive note using the subjective objective assessment plan (SOAP) method, although some advocate the subjective objective opinion options assessment agreed plan (SOOOAAP) technique. Remember that lawsuits often occur years after patient treatment and the doctor may not even recall seeing the patient. In such cases, patient records will often be the best witness for the defense.

The essentials of good documentation should also include all the elements listed in Box 4 but should never include the following elements:

Personal (other than medical/dental) opinions
Speculation on causes of poor outcomes

Box 4. Essentials of good documentation

Required patient information

- Completed and signed patient medical and dental history form
- Radiographs (labeled and dated)
- Patient name, address, telephone number, date of birth, and age
- Physician's name and telephone number
- Emergency contact information

Patient visit note

- Date and time at each entry
- Note of review of medical and allergic history (initial encounter)
- SOAP note
- Drugs administered to patient
- Prescription given to patient
- Instructions given to patient
- Referrals made and referrals or instructions not followed
- Telephone conversation with patient and physician
- Cancellation/new appointment
- Laboratory tests ordered
- Results of laboratory tests or consultants' reports

Derogatory statements about the patient or his/her family
Professional disputes
Financial payments or plans (keep in separate part of record)
Reference to legal actions, attorneys, or risk-management activities

Drug sensitivities and allergies

A complete medical history must also include a review of past reactions to medications and a history of medication allergies. Allergy alert stickers or clearly marked alerts must be placed directly on the patient's record for immediate identification of the patient's allergic history, thereby avoiding potential serious complications.

Handwriting

Malpractice cases have been lost purely because of the poor appearance of a patient's chart; as some people say, "A sloppy chart means a sloppy doctor." Therefore, attention to handwriting and legibility are vital to good care and a positive judgment. If a doctor has difficulty in this area, dictation and transcription services and computerized recording systems are available.

Documentation of telephone encounters

The use of the telephone (and the Internet) expands the dentist's practice capabilities and the risks; therefore, documenting telephone conversations takes on a significant importance, similar to any direct patient contact.

Telephone patient discussions relevant to clinical care often occur after hours, especially in a surgical or endodontic practice. Clinical advice, recommendations, and prescriptions are often prescribed and need to be documented in the patient's chart; a patient who initiates a lawsuit years later can allege that anything and everything was discussed on the telephone, and will have telephone records proving a call was made and received. Because of the length of time that has passed, the treating dentist without proper documentation will most likely not recall the conversation or how it occurred.

Documentation should also include any follow-up calls made to check on the status of the patient's condition following a surgical procedure or lengthy dental work.

Similarly, staff must be trained to screen telephone calls and put through those calls that are significant, important, and truly emergent, because patients are sensitive to the issue of emergency contacts.

Ownership of records

Dentists are required to maintain their dental records for a given period of years, depending on state statute. New York State Department of Education regulations require records to be stored for 6 years after last treatment in adults, and for children, until 2.5 years past the age of majority (ie, until age 23.5) or more (if treatment was rendered from age 18 and on). But the recommended and safest approach is to keep records forever because professional discipline cases have no statute of limitations.

Retired dentists are bound to keep records for 6 years minimum and longer for minors. Because of variance in state laws, it is important for all dentists to contact their state dental society for specific state regulations. The dentist owns the patient radiographs and records, and originals are never to be relinquished to anyone except in response to a subpoena. Copies are to be released only with the written authorization of the patient or legal guardian. It is appropriate to charge patients for copies (75 cents per page) and a reasonable rate for radiographs and study models. A dentist cannot deny any patient's request for copies because of unpaid bills.

If an employee dentist leaves the practice to begin his/her own practice, the employer dentist has the absolute obligation to provide a copy of a patient's record on written request by the patient.

Medical/dental records must always be well secured and protected from theft, damage, or destruction. Original records must never be removed from the doctor's control without a court order; other than this, they should never leave the office.

Electronic records must be backed up on a regular basis and stored securely. Medical/dental records should be stored for many years per state requirements and when disposed of, careful attention should be paid to patient confidentiality. Shredding or incineration are the methods of choice and are the ones used most often for destroying patient records.

Follow-up system

Failure to follow up patients for pathology, infection, pain, and so forth, can lead to the patient's getting lost in the system, and possible litigation. The dentist should always review consultant reports (radiology, oral pathology, and so forth) before filing them in the patient's chart and should make a note of the findings in the patient's record.

A mechanism should be instituted in a busy office that will signal the staff to call or write to those patients who missed a follow-up appointment, so that the dentist can put final closure on any outstanding issue and will not be rudely informed 6 months later of the patient's severe adverse outcome that has ultimately led to a lawsuit.

Referral for treatment

Dentists need to be critically aware that negligence not only is defined by acts of commission but also includes acts of omission. Failure to refer a patient to a specialist for consultation or treatment in a timely manner is considered negligent behavior and will lead to a malpractice situation if any poor outcome results from this delay of referral. The dentist must ask him/herself the following questions:

Is the treatment beyond my capability?
Is the level of complications high, and can I treat those complications?
Can I capably perform the procedure? Do I have the proper training and experience?
Is the patient comfortable with my performing the procedure?

If the patient refuses referral

1. Document referral in chart.
2. Explain in detail the risks to the patient for not following through with treatment.
3. Record in the patient's record that you informed the patient of his/her problem and reasons for referral to the specialist.

Abandonment

Health care providers are not legally obligated, nor do they have a duty, to treat all patients who enter their office, unless they agree to do so. This statement is generally true, but dentists on call for their hospital emergency medicine department, or who are on managed care panels, may be bound by hospital bylaws or state laws to accept all such patients; inquiries to their hospital medical board or managed care program should be made if one decides not to treat such a patient. However, once a doctor–patient relationship is established, treatment continues until 1) the patient's condition no longer warrants attention, 2) the patient leaves the practice, 3) a mutual doctor–patient decision is made to terminate care, or 4) the doctor chooses to end the relationship.

Financial disagreement should not have a bearing on the doctor–patient relationship. Those patients who are not compliant with instructions that may jeopardize the outcome of care, who continuously fail to meet their appointments, or who are verbally or physically abusive to the doctor or staff may be discharged from care. Certain legal protocols, however, should be followed when terminating the doctor–patient relationship to avoid charges of patient abandonment:

- The doctor should send a letter to the patient by certified mail informing the patient of his/her intention to end the doctor–patient relationship. The doctor does not need to state a reason, but one should avoid stating "incompatibility" as a reason or discussing any personal issues in the letter.
- The doctor should be sure that the patient's condition at the time of termination is stable and not emergent.
- The patient should be given the address or name of a colleague who has agreed to see the patient, the name of a dental school, or the dental society referral services number.
- The patient's missed appointments should be documented. Failure to comply with office recommendations of care, and any abusive behavior, should be recorded in the patient's chart.
- The doctor should inform the patient that all the records will be available for transfer.
- The doctor should inform the patient that he/she will be available for emergency care for a 2- to 3-month period, depending on the demographics and the patient's ability to find a new dentist.

Trends in dental professional liability claims

The American Dental Association's Council on Member's Insurance and Retirement Programs recently (in 2005) completed a comprehensive survey of 15 insurance companies that underwrite dental professional liability insurance, and who cover 104,557 dentists. The survey results presented here are valuable to the dental community in revealing trends in malpractice allegations and opportunity for improvement in the quality of dental care provided.

Record-keeping issues

Professional liability insurance companies have long asserted that errors or inadequacies in patient records prevent them from successfully defending some dentists against unfounded allegations of malpractice. To identify the area in greatest need of improvement in record keeping, the council sought to determine the relative severity of various errors. The following question was posed to the insurers, with respect to general practitioners and specialists: "Please indicate the degree to which your company has noted the following types of problems with its insured patients' records (whether or not the problem was a primary cause of a paid claim)." To quantify the responses to this subjective question, a value of 10 was assigned to any problem that was indicated as being "very common." If a problem was "fairly common," it was assigned a value of 5. If the insurer said that the problem was "not common," it was assigned a value of 0. The average scores for each problem, reflecting the opinions of 14 insurers weighed equally, are listed in Table 1.

These results indicate that, in the opinion of professional liability insurance companies, it is commonplace to find dentists who have presented claims who are not adequately documenting treatment plans, the patient's medical history, or an informed consent/refusal process. Whether this result is indicative of the need for improvement in record keeping among all dentists is conjectural. However, the American Dental Association Council believes all dentists should review their own record-keeping practices to identify whether any of the issues shown in the survey need to be addressed.

Communications issues

Another set of factors that can impact the ability of an insurer to defend a dentist against an unfounded allegation of malpractice is the quality of the communications between the dentist and the patient. To evaluate the frequency of problems in patient communications, the final part of the survey asked the insurers to answer the following question with respect to general practitioners and specialists: "Please indicate the degree to which your company has noted the following types of problems involving communications (whether or not the problem was a primary cause of a paid claim)." As with the previous question, a value of 10 was assigned to any problem that was indicated as being "very common," a value of 5 if the problem was "fairly common," and a value of 0 if the problem was "not common." The average scores for each problem, reflecting the opinions of 14 insurers weighed equally, are listed in Table 2.

The standout results to this question are the high scores assigned by insurers to the issue of intraprofessional criticisms and to claims filed in

Table 1
Insurers' views as to the frequency of various record-keeping errors

Type of error, in descending order of frequency	Average score[a]
Treatment plan is not documented	6.5
Health history is not clearly documented or updated regularly	6.1
Informed consent is not documented	5.9
Informed refusal is not documented	5.0
Assessment of patient is incompletely documented	4.9
Words, symbols, or abbreviations are ambiguous	4.9
Telephone conversations with patient are not documented	4.6
Treatment rendered is not clearly documented	4.5
Subjective complaints are not documented	4.1
Objective findings are incompletely documented	4.1
Treatment plan is not supported by documented subjective and objective findings	4.0
Reasons for deviation from the original treatment plan are not documented	3.9
Patient noncompliance or failed appointments are not documented	3.7
Records are not legible	3.7
Routine full-mouth periodontal probing is not documented	3.4
Records are insufficient, given the complexity of the issue	3.2
Postoperative instructions are not documented	3.2
Referral to, or consultation with, another practitioner or physician is not documented	2.8
Comments about the cost of treatment and the patient's payment history	2.6
Radiographs were inadequate for the procedure	2.3
Prescription orders are not documented	2.2
Deletions, additions, or corrections are not made properly	2.0
Risk management notations included in the chart	1.4
The name and relationship of the person who gave consent is not documented for minors or patients who are incapacitated	1.4
Records are altered	1.1
Records/radiographs are lost	.7
Records are not written in ink	.7
Record contains notations relating to discussions with an attorney or insurer regarding a possible malpractice lawsuit	.4
The chart contains critical or subjective personal comments about the patient	.4

[a] Scores were assigned as follows: very common, 10; fairly common, 5; not common, 0.

retaliation to billing disputes. They assigned higher scores, on average, to these issues than to other communications and record-keeping problems, which may indicate that some dentists need more guidance in handling these sensitive matters.

A third question was, "For your policyholders who are general practitioners, please indicate the approximate percentage of paid claims that included the allegations listed in Table 3."

Table 2
Insurers' views as to the frequency of various dentist–patient communication issues

Communication issue	Average score[a]
Critical comments of the insured's work made to a patient by another dentist or dentists	7.7
Professional liability claim filed in retaliation for a billing dispute or collection problem	6.7
Lack of, or poor, communication between a primary dentist and a specialist	4.1
Reliance on a signed release form in lieu of a discussion with a patient to obtain informed consent	2.0
Lack of, or poor, communication between a dentist and a physician	1.5
Professional liability claim filed subsequent to a peer review hearing	1.2
Inappropriate comments made to patients by dental office staff	0.9
Lack of, or poor, communication between a dentist and a patient's pharmacy	<0.1
Poor communication between dentist and patient	<0.1

[a] Scores were assigned as follows: very common, 10; fairly common, 5; not common, 0.

The standout results to this question are the percentage of claims alleging failure to diagnose and the percentage alleging inappropriate procedures. The conditions that were allegedly undiagnosed, and the types of treatment that most frequently involved allegations of inappropriate procedures, might be the subject of future surveys.

Table 3
Allegations involved in paid claims

Allegation	Paid claims that included this allegation
Failure to diagnose	12.3%
Inappropriate procedure	11.7%
Failure to obtain informed consent	8.5%
Failure to refer	5.4%
Treatment of wrong tooth	4.8%
Anesthesia complications	2.9%
Poor communications with patient's specialist	2.7%
Failure to treat medically compromised patients appropriately	2.6%
Equipment failure	2.4%
Alteration of treatment records	2.3%
Inadequate heath history	2.0%
Failure to detect tumor/cancer	1.6%
Employee performance causing claim	1.4%
Abandonment	1.3%
Incorrect prescriptions	1.2%
No radiograph, or incomplete radiograph	1.2%
Assault/excessive force	.8%
Sexual harassment	.4%
Doctors made guarantees for success of procedures	.3%
Breach of confidentiality	0%
Other	34.2%
Total	100%

Summary

Litigation and malpractice suits are a part of everyday life in medical/dental practice. The astute clinician must be as diligent in risk-reduction management and strategies as he/she is in practicing excellent dentistry. Good patient communication, rapport, and excellent documentation are the keys to minimizing, and possibly eliminating future lawsuits.

References

[1] Deegan AE. Selected readings in oral and maxillofacial surgery, risk prevention for oral and maxillofacial surgeons. Vol 6. Dallas (TX): The University of Texas Southwestern Medical Center at Dallas. p. 1.
[2] AAOMS National Insurance Company 6133 N River Road, Rosemont, IL 60001.
[3] The advisors. AAOMS Risk Management Journal 1987;2(3):7–9.
[4] Hycke LI, Hycke MM. Characteristics of potential plaintiffs in malpractices litigation. Ann Intern Med 1994;120:792.

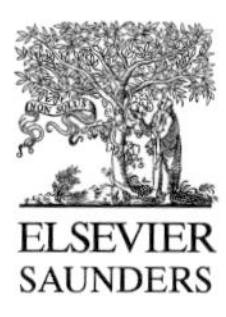
ELSEVIER
SAUNDERS

Dent Clin N Am 52 (2008) 579–603

THE DENTAL
CLINICS
OF NORTH AMERICA

Stress Management in the Difficult Patient Encounter

Stanley Bodner, PhD[a,b,*]

[a]*Department of Social Science, Adelphi University-University College, 1 South Avenue, Garden City, NY 11530, USA*

[b]*1805 East 17th Street, Brooklyn, NY 11229-2912, USA*

It is almost axiomatic that dentistry be viewed as a stress-laden profession. Rada and Johnson-Leong [1] cogently imply that the sources of stress for the practicing dentist derive from two key factors: the dentist's office or working environment and the dentist's personality, makeup, and lifestyle. Some dentists experience enormous, and what appears to be unmitigated, stress during the course of the day. These dentists find it difficult to contain their emotions and are predisposed to succumb to inner feelings of stress when encountering either demanding patients or challenging cases. At times, some dentists may perceive that some of their own staff members tend to sabotage what they consider to be proper office practice. In some instances, the stress experienced by the dentist stems from fear of the litigious-prone patient.

The already existing psychologic conditions of some dentists are exacerbated with the passage of time; or the dentist may develop anxiety-related disorders, depressive symptoms, professional "burnout," or other clinical syndromes. When burnout sets in, the dentist feels emotionally, and even physically, exhausted. Often, the latter state is accompanied by the unfolding of a cynical purview toward patients and staff, and self-perceptions of incompetence may also evolve. Consultation with a mental health professional is imperative when professional burnout defines the dentist's psyche.

The intent of this article is to spotlight aspects of the dentist's day-to-day challenges which might contribute to acute or prolonged feelings of stress. A special focus is on unique patient personae that govern certain patient

* Department of Social Science, Adelphi University-University College, 1 South Avenue, Garden City, NY 11530.

E-mail address: stanbodner@aol.com

doi:10.1016/j.cden.2008.02.012 **dental.theclinics.com**

behaviors which, in turn, may account for the stress experienced by the dentist. Coping techniques and strategies designed to reduce such stress are discussed. The concluding segment of the article presents an overview of stress management techniques that are offered as a means of promoting more effective coping strategies and, ultimately, as a pathway to using lifestyle changes that will serve to augment the dentist's quality of life.

Rather than offer a list of "do's" and "don'ts" in the management of the so-called "difficult" patient, this article attempts to alert the practitioner as to what perceptions or traits harbored by the dentist lead to his/her perception that a patient is "difficult"; what characteristics are inherent within the patient that make his/her behavior difficult for the dentist to deal with; and how stress engendered by the encounter may be minimized.

The first section of the article provides an overview, or primer, that serves to highlight the physical and psychologic underpinnings of stress. A discussion follows that presents the correlational links between the experience of stress and the development and maintenance of certain health-related disorders. Stress-related health disorders are the products of the "wear and tear" of cumulative incidents and experiences the dentist encounters in his/her day-to-day practice. The perception of difficulty should be targeted for alteration and adjustment, with the net effect of reducing stress.

The nature of stress

Stress is an inevitable fact of life. Having stress is an experience that cannot be eschewed by the living. Perhaps stress should be viewed as the price we pay for being alive.

When an individual experiences, through physical sensation or psychologic perception, a need for a sudden adjustment or response, he/she might perceive the event as being stressful. The demands placed on the individual to adjust in the face of a dynamic situation may set into motion physical and internal reactions and sensations. The term "stress" has generally encompassed the adjustive demands or press placed on the individual and that individual's biologic response to those demands [2].

Stress is experienced by the individual as a physical or psychologic tension that places his/her system into some level of disequilibrium. The perceived experience of stress should spur the individual to adjust to the attending challenges that the stressor or stressors engender. The efforts the individual undertakes to escape the tensions stimulated by stressors are often referred to as coping strategies or coping mechanisms. Neufeld [3] conceptualizes stress as the consequence of inadequate or inferior coping skills or coping interventions. He suggests that the experience of stress and the attempts undertaken to cope with the felt stress are intertwined in an almost inverse fashion; the more efficient one's coping skills, the less one's perceived sense of stress is expected to be. Selye [4,5] dichotomized the concept of stress by differentiating between the tensions that arise when positive life events demanding adjustments occur (eustress) and the adjustments undertaken in the face of perceived negative life events (distress). Being conferred the status of valedictorian might stimulate eustress; having an insurance company delay payment for an approved, complicated dental procedure may engender a feeling of distress. Whether the individual faces eustress or distress, he/she has to draw on his/her capacity to implement successful coping mechanisms; nonetheless, a cumulative history of distressful experiences has been correlated with the development of deleterious health consequences.

Butcher and colleagues [2] point out three categories of stressors: frustrations, conflicts, and pressures. Frustrations can derive from either internally perceived or externally perceived obstacles, which can serve to thwart or stymie an individual's goals or plans. A dentist, for instance, who cares little about engaging in certain procedures or, perhaps, views him/herself as unskilled in certain techniques endures frustrations springing from internal factors; not being permitted to expand a dental practice because of inadequate capital represents an external or an environmental source of frustration. Conflicts arise when an individual is presented or confronted with two concurrent and vying needs, motives, demands, or plans of action. Pursuing or fulfilling one's need or plan of action precludes fulfillment of the other or competing need (opportunity cost). This phenomenon dovetails nicely with Festinger's [6] classic description of cognitive dissonance. For example, an established general dentist who wishes to pursue advanced training in orthodontics or in some other specialized training but weighs this path against the compromises to personal and professional obligations that such training will require experiences internal angst or conflict. One's experience of stress may originate not only from frustrating or conflicting situations but also from the pressure to reach or meet particular sought-after goals or perceived imposed expectations. When pressure is experienced, the individual may feel compelled to work harder, longer, or more intensely than he/she normally would, which might overload his/her existing coping skills and lead to a concentrated experience of stress and even such maladaptive or self-destructive behaviors as self-medicating through drug ingestion to escape pressure. A dentist who expands his/her practice simply to please his/her spouse (external pressure) or because it will lead to greater recognition from colleagues (internal pressure) might experience prolonged stress as a consequence of these ill-conceived undertakings.

Physiologic aspects of stress

Whether stress stems from a biologic stimulus or from perceived psychologic press that demands a response or an adjustment from the individual, several physiologic processes, including the release of stress hormones, are activated. To appreciate why the stress we experience leads to sympathetic nervous responses such as tachycardia, increased perspiration, muscle contractions (especially in the trapezius and frontalis areas), the psychologic perception of apprehension and the release of corticosteroids and epinephrine and norepinephrine, one has to understand the stress response first described by Cannon [7] and dubbed the "fight or flight" response. This stress response, or alarm reaction, directly results from the activation of the sympathetic division of the nervous system and from select glands in the endocrine system that are sensitive to stress. When the individual perceives an event as stressful, the adrenal glands, mediated by the pituitary gland, stimulate the production of corticosteroids and catecholamines, which activate the sympathetic response, alluded to earlier. Specifically, Selye [4,5] pointed out that the anterior pituitary–adrenal cortex system is activated when stressors are perceived by the individual. Adrenocorticotropic hormone, released from the anterior pituitary, stimulates, in turn, the release of glucocorticoids from the adrenal cortex. The glucosteroids engender within the individual many of the sensations experienced during the stress response [8,9]. In fact, the amount of circulating glucosteroids serves as a physiologic marker of the individual's stress level. At the same time that the adrenal cortex stimulates the release of glucocorticoids in the system, the sympathetic response of the adrenal medulla releases higher levels of epinephrine and norepinephrine [10].

Selye [4,5] advanced the concept of the general adaptation syndrome (GAS), which arises in the face of extended or extensive stress. Selye proposed that the GAS sets into motion an alarm response that does not cease until the energy turned on by the stress response is exhausted. Any perceived stressor, whether it is an internal response such as inhibition of inflammation, or a response to environmental stressors, such as a letter arriving from the Internal Revenue Service or a dentist interacting with a difficult patient, may set off the initial stage of the alarm reaction of the GAS. The alarm reaction, in turn, concurrently activates the sympathetic division of the autonomic nervous system and the segment of the endocrine system that responds to stress, which, again, is the essence of the fight or flight response. Although this response is functional during an actual or genuine threat to the individual, it is not functional when a situation bears no actual threat. Moreover, when an actual threat to the individual is removed, the parasympathetic division of the autonomic nervous system takes over and mediates a moderating influence, effectively halting the stress response. However, when personal and professional demands and stressors seem overwhelming and unremitting, we tend to adapt to a living pattern in which the stress alarm remains activated. In time, with the continued hyperarousal of the sympathetic nervous system, the individual may succumb to a stress-related illness or disorder.

In describing the GAS, Selye explained that when a stressor is experienced in prolonged fashion, the individual eventually enters into a phase of adaptation referred to as the resistance stage. During this stage, the endocrine system continues to emit stress hormones and sympathetic nervous system responses remain highly activated, notwithstanding the removal of the perceived threat. That is, our stress response remains at high alert when it should not. In further applying the GAS model, the individual will eventually reach an exhaustion stage, in which bodily resources are depleted and, by default, the parasympathetic division of the autonomic nervous system takes over. Despite the operations of the GAS, if the individual perceives that certain stressors serve as an ever-present threat (eg, work or monetary pressures, anticipation of difficult dental procedures or patients), the individual may be at risk for diseases of adaptation, such as heart disease. Cohen and colleagues [11] emphasize that the buildup of cortical steroids in the system may account for why prolonged stress can contribute to the development of stress-related disorders and other issues. Although corticosteroids have usefulness in assisting the body cope with the physical aspects of stress, frequent cortical steroid deposits into the system will eventually debilitate the immune system because they tend to inhibit antibody protection, rendering the individual prey to opportunistic diseases [12–15].

One can anticipate that the dental practitioner who experiences frequent psychologic stressors, including dreading interaction with difficult patients, will tend to have increased levels of glucocorticoids, epinephrine, and norepinephrine. Such elevations in stress hormones are linked to the promotion of an array of physical disorders [16]. Research has even shown that the experience of presurgical anxiety, especially of an exaggerated nature, has been linked to slow postsurgical recuperation and wound healing [17,18].

The interplay between psychologic stress and somatic disorders

We have significantly distanced ourselves from the dualistic notion, espoused by Descartes during the 17th century, that the mind and body are distinct and separate spheres. Much research is available that relates the impact of psychic stress to bodily dysregulation and illness. The diathesis-stress model has been posited as a theory designed to elucidate the mind–body relationship as it impacts the development or course of disease. A diathesis is conceived as a biologic or genetic predisposition, propensity, or vulnerability that places the individual at risk for falling prey to a specific disorder or disease syndrome. This theory further assumes that the burgeoning of a disorder hinges on the type and intensity of the stressors the individual encounters or sustains. The stressor or stressors that the individual experiences may run the gamut from prenatal or early developmental influences, physical or psychologic trauma, significant illness, familial pressures or dysfunction, the death of significant persons, working in an inhospitable environment, to, for the dentist, engaging a difficult or noncompliant patient.

The diathesis theory further asserts that an individual who harbors a diathesis for a specific disease or disorder may escape the illness if the degree of stress to which the individual is subjected is kept to a minimum, especially through applying effective coping strategies or techniques. Notwithstanding this point, it is also the case that the more forceful or vigorous the diathesis, the lower the level of stress needed to stimulate the manifestation of the disorder or dysfunctionality. The diathesis-stress theory has been presented frequently as a significant factor in the development of clinical depression [19,20]. Lewinsohn and colleagues [19] point out that the diathesis-stress model does not solely limit itself to biogenic factors; psychologically based diathesis is believed to be instrumental in accounting for the genesis of certain disorders during stressful life periods. Specifically, psychologic diatheses such as dogmatically adhering to irrational or faulty cognitions, having an anxious or inadequate personality structure, or experiencing emotional upheavals such as divorce, death, or familial strife, places the individual at greater risk for exogenous or reactive depression, which, in turn, can serve to compromise the immune system's integrity.

The experience of prolonged stress has been closely linked to many physical or somatic disorders. It may not be the case that a particular psychologic disturbance such as depression or an anxiety-related disorder is causative to a disease process; nevertheless, psychologic factors often serve as contributory factors in the formation or exacerbation of physical disorders. For example, extant research presents evidence that stress can give rise to chronic headaches because it stimulates contractions to the muscles of the neck, scalp, face, and shoulders [21]. In fact, when electromyogram biofeedback is used in stress management programs to treat nonmigraine or tension-related headaches, sensors are attached to either the frontalis or trapezius areas because both emit increased microvolts of energy when the individual feels tense. Sorbi and colleagues [22] concluded that the cumulative experiences of so-called "minor," albeit irritating, life stressors, combined with either a "quick-trigger" excitable or irascible temperament, or even sleep deprivation, may serve as significant factors in the development of different types of migraine headaches.

Cardiovascular disorders, such as coronary heart disease and hypertension, are tied to psychologic disturbances caused by stress and the individual's characterological makeup. The intense or hard-driving lifestyle of the type A personality, with his/her concomitant characteristics of aggressive competitiveness and an inner or outward sense of hostility, is thought to be more prone than his/her non–type A (type B) counterpart to the development of cardiovascular disorders [23–25].

In more recent times, Denollet [26], through extensive research, was able to isolate the specific damaging emotions inherent within the type A personality that appear most linked to coronary heart disease and hypertension. Thus, the type A was refined into the current type D personality. Individuals who rank high on Denollet's type D (distress) scale, especially by endorsing items suggestive of high levels of anxiety, hostility, and hopelessness, have a more than 400% greater probability of experiencing a cardiac attack or death within 6 to 9 months of undergoing angioplasty with stent placements, compared with non–type D peers who have received similar cardiac treatment.

Krantz and colleagues [27] suggested that the demands of stressful occupations or professions (eg, dentistry) can be tempered by such personality traits as psychologic hardiness or flexibility. A wholesome professional outlook can, thus, moderate the effects of occupational stress and, in consequence, can lower the risk of developing coronary heart disease. Jorgensen and colleagues [28] found that high levels of anxiety, anger, and depression, which are emotions often experienced during periods of stress, are correlated with the incidence of hypertension, a precursor of heart disease.

Although Helicobacter pylori (*H Pylori*) bacterium has been implicated in the development of many gastric ulcers, much evidence exists that supports the hypothesis that stress serves as a contributory factor or plays a maintenance role in the development, exacerbation, or perpetuation of a peptic ulcer [29]. Thus, even in instances in which a bacterium is thought to give rise to an individual's ulcer, stress may impede the healing process in the mucosal lining of the stomach or duodenum.

Although it might be dubious to advance the notion that stress is directly linked to the formation of malignant cancer cells in systems or organs, evidence is persuasive that psychologic states of depression may compromise the efficacy of the individual's immune system, which, in turn, can influence the proliferation of cancer cells [30]. Sklar and Anisman [31] actually present evidence from animal and human studies that unchecked stress might serve as a contributor to the proliferation of tumors. Of course, if such research findings can be held up consistently, it would imply that proper stress management could serve to promote remission.

Research provides evidence that acute stress (eg, being in an anxious state when engaged in a difficult patient encounter) or chronic stress (eg, ongoing marital conflict) can negatively affect the integrity of the immune system. Prolonged or unmitigated stress may hamper phagocytosis, or the process by which phagocytes are able to engulf foreign microorganisms such as viruses. Some correlational studies suggest an existing linkage between sustained stress and susceptibility to infectious disease [32–34].

The foregoing segment essentially serves as a brief overview of some suspected consequences of long-term, or unchecked, stress. What follows serves as a "spotlight" on the stress that the dental practitioner experiences in dealing with different types of challenging patients, with an eye on better management of the stress.

What makes certain patients difficult to treat or interact with? Why are some patients noncompliant with the proposed treatment plan that was explained with due time and effort? How is the dentist best able to cope with the stresses and strains of an obstinate or incommodious patient? How does the dentist proceed with necessary treatment that a patient may needlessly turn into an Augean task?

The essence of cognitive behavioral psychology hinges on the basic tenet that it is not the "things, people, and places" we come across in life that disturb us; rather, it is the way we perceive or react to them. If we alter these perceptions, our feelings and actions become more rational. As we approach our challenges more calmly and realistically, we will discover that our reactions to the vicissitudes of life are experienced with less stress and struggle.

What makes a patient difficult? Some common explanations include:

- Patient fear or anger
- Faulty attributions or projected motivations or characteristics placed onto the practitioner
- Inappropriate hostility displaced onto the dentist
- Misinterpretation of what treatment is needed, or poor provider–patient communications leading to poor patient comprehension of treatment
- Ingrained patient issues with perceived authority figures
- Lack of patient trust in the practitioner
- Clash between the inherent respective personality traits of the patient and dentist
- Patient's perception of the dentist's lack of sympathy or caring regarding the patient's plight

The difficult patient encounter

Concerning ourselves with the so-called "difficult patient" actually places the focus in the wrong place. What is difficult is the relationship, per se, between the patient and the dentist, and, for treatment to have the chance to succeed, the patient–dentist relationship requires change or improvement. Studies undertaken in the medical profession estimate that as many as 15% to 25% of the patient population are viewed as difficult [35].

When attempting to discern what contributes to a difficult patient–dentist encounter, it is necessary to ascertain which patient and practitioner characteristics contribute to the challenging interaction.

Patient characteristics

The following patient behaviors, perceptions, or traits appear to contribute to difficult encounters:

- A patient who demands that treatment should proceed according to his/her understanding or predilection
- A patient who is manipulative with respect to the dentist's or staff's time either through prolonging his/her visit or by cajoling staff for accommodations not provided to others

- A patient who presents with vaguely expressed dental complaints
- A patient who has dental complaints that have no biologic grounding or physical basis (somatization)
- A patient who does not follow through with prior recommendations, or is otherwise noncompliant
- A patient who minimizes the gravity or severity of his/her dental problems
- A patient who provides "socially desirable" responses to questions posed by the dentist, thereby minimizing the true extent of his/her dental issues or degree of treatment compliance
- A patient who assigns or transfers complete responsibility of care and treatment follow-up to the dentist
- A patient who presents a multiplicity of complaints, many perhaps irrelevant, that stymie diagnosis or treatment focus
- A patient who "straps" the dentist with his/her personal problems, confusing dental therapy with psychotherapy
- The addicted patient who views the dentist as a ready source for benzodiazepine or opioid prescriptions
- The chronic pain patient whose dental complaints tend to be diffuse or ambiguous and for whom sundry modifications in procedures need to be contemplated
- A patient who clearly presents with either subtle or frank psychopathology, ranging from schizophrenia to bipolar to anxiety-related disorders
- A malingering patient who is actively involved or seriously weighing the filing of a disability or workers' compensation claim

If the dentist responds to any of these patient behaviors or presentations with anger, resentment, avoidance, dysphoria, deflation, or a sense of futility or helplessness, he/she will experience some level of stress and will view the interaction as difficult. It is clear that the most important first step is for the dentist to be cognizant as to why he/she perceives the patient encounter as difficult, and then he/she needs to use an appropriate coping strategy. This strategy might require a conscious effort to alter the perception of the patient or experience, effectively rendering the interaction with the patient as less stressful. Elder and colleagues [36], in a study surveying physicians on how they manage difficult patients, found that those who mentally braced and prepared themselves by taking inventory of their personal attitudes, biases, and expectations (in tandem, if need be, with the use of breathing and relaxation exercises) were better able to handle such difficult patient encounters.

Medical studies have shown that difficult, demanding, or troubled patients may actually be manifesting some level of psychopathology, which may range from mild to moderate to severe intensity [37–39]. Highly anxious patients, for example, tend to express multiple complaints or might comment that the dentist or his/her staff is inattentive or unresponsive to his/her needs, which, in fact, is not the case. Another subset of patients may be diagnosed with a personality disorder and will present with such intractable, characterological issues as manipulativeness, obduracy, dependency, or narcissism. Bodner [40] has previously addressed the psychologic aspects of chronic pain patients and the various personality traits and styles they adopt which parallel, in many respects, patients who engender difficult encounters.

Dentist characteristics

The dental practitioner may be facing several pressures or external stressors that serve as a source of ongoing tension. The dentist may also possess personality traits that predispose him/her to color his/her perceptions, leading to the assessment that a particular encounter is a difficult one.

In the following examples, the perspective of the dentist is taken to better understand how a particular encounter may be experienced as difficult:

- The dentist who views a talkative patient as being too distracting as he/she performs a dental procedure
- The dentist who feels the pressures of time constraints and prefers an efficient use of time who may view a patient as difficult if the interaction is somehow not conforming to time strictures
- The dentist who is overburdened with work and can't seem to "catch up" with his/her schedule
- As in medicine [41], a dentist who may have been in practice for many years and may be subject to "burnout syndrome," leading to the perception of difficulties in a patient encounter when, objectively speaking, neither the encounter nor the patient is difficult at all
- The dentist who cannot satisfactorily ameliorate the presenting complaint and may view him/herself as incompetent
- The dentist who feels that a patient is taking advantage of office services by expecting extraoffice services
- The dentist who perceives that the patient wishes to direct the treatment plan
- The dentist who perceives that a personality mismatch with the patient exists, priming the practitioner to perceive the patient in a negative light

Patient personas that tend to contribute to difficult encounters

A discussion follows regarding the personas that contribute to strained dentist–patient interactions. The psychologic dynamics that can, perhaps, account for the reason why a patient presents as either angry or anxious, or that in other ways contribute to a difficult encounter, will now be examined, followed by a section designed to provide useful strategies that should serve to mitigate the stress or tension of such difficult interactions. The discussion on coping techniques concludes with overall stress management strategies that the dentist can use either within the office setting (if feasible) or as enhancers for improved quality of life.

The angry patient

A patient can present with an angry or hostile disposition for several reasons, the basis of which may not be readily manifest. Although, at times, the patient may actually display anger toward the dentist, the anger may also be directed toward office staff. Patients who perceive the dentist as being unsympathetic, uncaring, disengaged, distracted, or even flippant with respect to the presenting dental complaint can be expected to engender the patient's ire. Office staff who are perceived as rude, unresponsive, or unreceptive to questions or accommodations, or who communicate in either an abrupt or a condescending fashion, can create an atmosphere which stimulates patient anger. Staff are viewed as an extension of the practitioner, and patient anger that has as its basis poor staff treatment may, in turn, be projected onto the dentist. The source or genesis giving rise to the patient's anger may escape the dentist's awareness, leading him/her to conclude erroneously that the patient is just an angry person.

In several instances, patient anger bears no relation whatsoever to the dentist's or the staff's treatment or regimen. Patients arrive at the dentist's office with their unique histories, lifestyles, experiences, and perceptions. If a patient presents an angry demeanor replete with negative verbal and nonverbal communications, it is possible that they are beset with personal or interpersonal conflicts or issues and their anger is being discharged or displaced in the office setting.

Managing the stress that the angry patient engenders

To respond to a patient's angry communication with a defensive posture is wholly inappropriate. Professionalism dictates that the dentist attempt to understand the basis of the anger. Defensiveness, counterarguing, and confrontation will almost always serve to escalate the situation and exacerbate the tension already felt. McCullough and colleagues [42] describe the BATHE technique and encourage this approach as a means toward reducing the stress engendered when facing a difficult encounter. At the outset, the practitioner should assess the background (B) of the situation to ascertain the nature of the problem presented by the patient and the consequent affect (A) or emotion attached to the presenting problem. The next step is for the practitioner to triage the problem that disturbs or troubles (T) the patient most. This step should be the dentist's focus. The practitioner then needs to determine how the patient is handling (H) the problem. The final step in interacting with a difficult patient is to be able to communicate empathy (E), which transmits to the patient a congruent understanding of the patient's problem.

Essary and Symington [43] recommend that in applying the BATHE technique to the treatment of a patient displaying anger, the following approach should be undertaken: At "B," or when assessing the background, the patient is encouraged to discuss with the practitioner what he/she is experiencing today. In determining the intensity of the affect ("A") of anger, the patient may relate that he/she is upset by the amount of waiting time, but may also provide information that sheds light on external factors that may be contributing to his/her anger. In ascertaining the "T," or what is troubling the patient that led to the appointment, the nature of the actual dental problem will become more crystallized. The lengthy wait, combined with the concern connected to the presenting dental complaint, may provide the dentist with necessary insight into the patient's perception of the experience. The dentist can then convey empathetic understanding that is compatible with the patient's current level of upset, discomfort, or even fear.

It is a reasonable expectation that if the practitioner can somehow mollify the patient's anger, the dentist's own stress (if any) will also be lessened. Devoting a few moments to allow for venting, or acknowledging the possibility of some legitimacy or justification for the patient's feelings of anger, may prove useful in moving the necessary treatment along. Thus, acknowledging to the patient, "You seem to be upset...do you wish to talk about it?" may give some insight as to the patient's target of anger, be it office staff, office routine or policy, the outside environment, or the dentist him/herself. Securing some level of understanding as to what is promoting the patient's anger places the dentist in the position to assuage or mitigate the anger. Presumably, with genuine expressions of sympathy or empathy, smoother treatment delivery can ensue with, it is to be hoped, a patient more invested and cooperative with treatment. If a few moments of time provided to tamp down patient anger, treatment efficacy can be expected. Fernandez and Turk [44] have asserted that anger heightens the subjective perception of pain through the activation of the autonomic nervous system. If the dentist makes no attempt to gain insight into the patient's anger, dental care and recovery can be hampered. Burns and colleagues [45] have cogently pointed out that patient suppression of articulated anger is associated with compromised or inferior treatment results. If, notwithstanding the dentist's sincere attempts at understanding or even legitimizing the patient's right to be upset through appropriate expressions of sympathy or empathy, the patient still maintains his/her anger, it is appropriate to place the responsibility of treatment continuation onto the patient. No dentist or other professional is required to be subjected to wanton, misplaced, or exaggerated anger, nor should the continuation of such behavior be reinforced. The dentist would do well to learn stress reduction techniques such as progressive muscle relaxation (PMR) coupled with positive imagery, and applications in cognitive reframing, as outlined in the final section of this article.

The anxious patient

As discussed by the author elsewhere [18], anxiety can be conceptualized as the patient's experience of tension, which either can be situation specific and transient (a state), or can stem from a chronic, characterological aspect of the individual (ie, a definable characteristic of the patient's personality makeup [a trait]). The experience of anxiety and the anticipation of pain in an upcoming dental procedure can be interlaced with one another. Because both factors can impact the perceived level of discomfort and pain tolerance, and treatment compliance and cooperativeness, it is necessary to address the patient's level of anxiety before treatment intervention. Ploghaus and colleagues [46] found that when anxious patients, who were anticipating the experience of pain, underwent brain scanning by way of functional MRI, the medial frontal lobe, the insula, and the cerebellum appeared activated, and these sites are located proximally to brain regions responsible for regulating the pain experience. Ploghaus and colleagues further explain that the very anticipation of pain can influence mood, which serves to heighten the perception of pain. McCracken and colleagues [47,48], who have developed the Pain Anxiety Symptom Scale, highlight the fact that high levels of anxiety are associated with cognitive distortion or misperception of the pain experience; feelings of agitation; an obsessive-like focus and the anticipation of pain; difficulties in concentration; escape-avoidance behaviors with respect to treatment; regressive routines undertaken to evince reassurance from others; and misuse/abuse of medications, such as anxiolytics.

Managing the stress that the anxious patient engenders

Intuitively, one should expect that by effectively reducing a patient's anxiety level, a corresponding reduction in the dentist's tension level would also result. Johnston and Vogele's [49] meta-analysis focused on how to affect positive surgical outcomes; however, it also effectively shed light on how to reduce the anxiety that a patient sometimes experiences when facing a dental procedure. That is, if the dentist allocates some reasonable amount of time to discussing a procedure, most patients will have better mental preparation. When necessary, instruction in relaxation techniques and positive imagery could prove useful in inducing a positive psychologic frame, leading to smoother and more efficient procedures and outcomes. When a patient is better informed about treatment, he/she is more inclined to feel empowered and will likely be more resigned to accept and brace for unavoidable discomfort.

The demanding patient or "micromanager"

The patient who presents a demanding stance is, at some level, expressing anticipated disappointment or discontent with treatment quality, delivery, or practitioner competency. A patient who demands that certain diagnostic measures or specific procedural approaches be used may be making such demands because of a host of possible motivations. If the patient's expectations are that relief or the course of treatment should follow a particular path or timetable, and these expectations are not realized, the patient may experience a sense of entitlement that justifies assertiveness and demands, directing the dentist to be guided by the patient's preferences. In other instances, a patient's demands may be driven by either a family member's or a friend's negative experience with a "similar" dental complaint, leading the patient to direct the dentist's treatment plan to avoid a similar fate.

Often, if patient demands are disregarded or not addressed, the patient may form a mistaken inference that the dentist did not properly assess the dental complaint. In other instances, a patient may demand a certain intervention, procedure, or treatment be undertaken in expeditious fashion to avoid greater pain (whether or not this effectively will be the case). Other patients may act in a demanding fashion because recent dental treatment did not seem successful in alleviating a presenting dental complaint. Still others may demand that the dentist follow a specific course of treatment because he/she has become a litigant in a lawsuit or is in the process of hatching a workers' compensation or disability case.

Regardless of what serves as the underlying catalyst for a patient's demands, the dentist must ascertain the underlying motive fueling the specific demands.

Managing the demanding patient

When a patient adopts a demanding stance, the dentist's reaction may give rise to any of the following emotions or self-perceptions: feelings of incompetence; feelings of rejection; self-blame or guilt; or a feeling that the patient lacks a sense of gratitude or appreciation for sincere effort and caring. The dentist may lapse into a defensive posture, justifying the rationale for a chosen treatment path, which might, in the process, cloud professional judgment and compromise care.

In coping with the tension that might be engendered when interacting with a demanding patient, one needs to feel confident about one's developed skills and mastery. The approach recommended is akin to that suggested for handling the angry or anxious patient, and that is to be accepting of the patient's feelings or emotions expressed in the demand. Thus, an exploratory statement such as, "You seem upset," or, "You seem frustrated," might direct the patient to express his/her specific concerns. A few moments of explanation of the dentist's treatment plan or the alternative strategies that might be undertaken if needed, could not only prove to be an effective tension reducer for the patient and dentist but could also lead to greater patient cooperation and compliance.

Sufficient communication and the validation of patient feelings have no substitute. Such practice will generally lead to calmer and more effective treatment experiences. When necessary, the dentist should take a few private moments to compose him/herself through appropriate "self-talk," when the rigors of dealing with a demanding patient prove too challenging. Afterwards, the adoption of a nonjudgmental approach, with ample bilateral communication, will often mitigate the intensity of demands.

Haas and colleagues [50] emphasize that it is counterproductive to ignore a patient's demands. It does not make the nature of the difficulty evaporate. Arguing, or otherwise engaging the patient in a defensive manner, may convert the demands into expressions of anger. Additionally, being dismissive of patient demands can motivate the patient to persist in his/her demands. Being receptive to any appropriate suggestions usually makes for the most efficient treatment strategy in working with a demanding patient.

The noncompliant patient and treatment management considerations

Patients can exhibit levels of treatment noncompliance through various means. Patients can manifest a noncompliant disposition by arriving late for an appointment or even by being a no-show for a scheduled appointment.

Patients may also exhibit noncompliant behavior by not following through with the dentist's instructions for proper maintenance or follow-up care. Actually, it is good practice for the dentist to record in the patient's chart all forms of noncompliance. Any outreach made to the patient should also be recorded.

It behooves the dentist to attempt to ascertain the basis for the noncompliant behavior. In some instances, basic communication may have broken down because of poor comprehension or language difficulty or simply by the patient's feeling too intimidated to express to the dentist why treatment compliance may be too difficult. Noncompliant behavior may stem from dissatisfaction with prior treatment received. Generally, the dentist is better equipped to facilitate improved compliance through improved listening and communication techniques.

The addicted patient and treatment management considerations

Key considerations concerning the treatment and management of patients suspected of substance abuse or chemical dependence have been addressed by the author elsewhere [18]; some key elements are addressed in this discussion.

It is essential, at the outset, to discern the difference between the patient who is seeking palliative pain relief and the patient who engages in manipulative behavior to extract a prescription for narcotics from the dentist. It is advised practice to be parsimonious in dispensing opiate-based prescriptions. As in all cases, prescribing opioids is secondary to diagnosis and is only undertaken when relief of pain is necessary. With the addicted patient, the report of pain is typically exaggerated or feigned.

The patterns of behavior, complaints, or observations [51] shown in Box 1 serve as possible indicators that a patient may be physically dependent on a substance, or substances, requiring the practitioner to adopt a strictly cautious approach.

In addition to these indicators, addiction specifically tied to opiates (eg, heroin, oxycontin, oxycodone, and codeine) is strongly suspected when the patient presents the following symptoms: diaphoresis; rhinorrhea; lacrimation; yawning; and complaints of muscle aches, especially in the lower extremities.

Many sensitive biochemical screeners are available for when alcohol addiction is of concern, in addition to existing paper-and-pencil inventories/questionnaires that can be easily administered. Bodner [18] provides a survey of instruments elsewhere. Sometimes, if a patient who demands pain medication shows more concern about coping with the pain of a dental problem and lesser interest in the cause for such pain, the question of substance dependence might be considered. Such concerns should be addressed before treatment.

Steps for managing difficult dentist–patient encounters

The strategy and steps of self-analysis proposed and outlined here may prove to be a useful tool for managing aspects of the difficult patient

Box 1. Indications of possible substance abuse or chemical dependence

- Complaints of sleep difficulties (hyposomnia or hypersomnia)
- Reports of recent seizure activity
- Malnutrition, anorexia, or a wasting appearance, often with the presentation of a pale complexion
- Abnormal liver function, such as elevations in alanine aminotransferase and aspartate aminotransferase enzymes detected in blood chemistries
- Altered moods and affect, such as expressions of irritability, dysphoria, or diffuse anxiety
- Complaints of chronic pain that appear exaggerated or vague in nature
- Poor hygiene or slovenly appearance
- General restlessness, agitation, hyperkinetic behavior
- Dry mouth and other anticholinergic symptoms
- Complaints of nausea and vomiting
- Slurred speech
- Motor clumsiness, tremors, shuffling gait
- Cigarette burns on fingers or clothing
- Unexplained bruises or scratches on face or extremities

encounter. This strategy is based on an amalgam of clinical research and observations. Table 1 outlines a stepwise approach to the management of difficult clinician–patient encounters. An expanded discussion is also presented.

Discussion

Recognition of the practitioner's emotional reaction to a perceived difficult encounter

The dentist must recognize and accept that he/she is experiencing some level of stress or other negative emotional response such as anxiety or irritation as he/she initiates some treatment with a patient or an encounter that is perceived as difficult. Such self-cognizance and self-recognition allows the dentist to adopt a more appropriate approach to the presenting dental complaint. Effective self-monitoring/management hinges on the dentist's level of self-awareness with respect to negative emotional responses [52].

Identification of the basis for perceiving an encounter as difficult

Is it the patient acting in a certain manner that stimulates a negative reaction within the dentist? Is it, possibly, the dentist with his/her unique or peculiar perceptual slant or set of personality traits that leads to interpreting

Table 1
A stepwise approach in the management of difficult patient encounters

Step	Function/rationale
1. Recognition of the practitioner's emotional reaction to a perceived difficult encounter	The dental practitioner becomes cognizant of his/her own negative response to a perceived difficult encounter, leading to better self-management.
2. Identification of the basis for perceiving an encounter as difficult	This analytic step is designed to pinpoint specifically what gives rise to the perceived difficulty.
3. Attempts at achieving perceptual congruence between dentist and patient	This step is designed to bring dentist and patient expectations regarding treatment into better alignment.
4. Adoption of a collaborative approach with the patient	Collaboration with a patient enhances patient investment and commitment to dentist's treatment plan.
5. Implementation and use of effective communication skills	Use of empathic understanding minimizes negative patient emotions or projections (especially undue anxiety), which, in turn, tends to predispose patients to be cooperative with treatment and follow-up.
6. Boundary setting	As necessary, patient must yield to dentist's treatment judgment and office protocol.

certain encounters as difficult? Perhaps, objectively speaking, the dentist is facing a complex or formidable case? In any event, awareness of what precisely is difficult about an encounter is the sine qua non of better management.

Attempts to achieve perceptual congruence between dentist and patient

White and Keller [53], in their analysis of difficult clinician–patient relationships, emphasize that what contributes to perceived difficulty in the clinician–patient interaction is what they refer to as misaligned expectations, which relate to the mismatch (noncongruence) in respective role expectations between the patient and practitioner. At the onset of treatment, patients may expect a certain approach, treatment, or timeframe, whereas the clinician's expectation of the patient is unqualified acceptance of his/her professional judgment and methodology, which implies strict compliance with the treatment plan devised by the dentist. A lack of congruence or perceptual alignment in treatment or role expectations will lead to the perception of difficulty or stress experienced by the dentist and the patient.

Adoption of a collaborative approach

Partnering with the patient is a useful tool that can be used by the dentist to enhance patient cooperation, commitment to treatment, and compliance. By outlining the treatment plan with the patient before the first step, eliciting questions or suggestions from the patient, and arriving at a consensus for the steps that will be undertaken, a message of respect for the patient's feelings is transmitted. Once the patient registers concurrence with the proposed plan, a brief review of the steps (corresponding to the complexity of the case) will further reinforce the plan's rationale. This step need not require an inordinate amount of time, and it often has the consequence of enhancing treatment efficacy.

Use of effective communication skills

If the dentist could adopt the mental frame of the patient and endeavor to experience the encounter as the patient does, he/she would better comprehend patient anxiety, resistance, irritability, or noncompliance, should it arise. Empathic understanding entails the capacity to imagine or experience the feelings that another person is experiencing, including his/her pain or distress [54]. The capacity for empathy is central to a good working clinician–patient relationship [55]. In Elder and colleagues' [36] survey of how practitioners effectively manage difficult patients, empathy is held to be the key, with an emphasis on focusing on the patient's emotions while imparting compassion blended with professional firmness. Empathic understanding with genuine expressions such as, "I hear anxiety in your voice," allows the patient to express why he/she is anxious, which, in turn, gives the dentist the opportunity to allay anxiety. Feedback is a necessary component in an empathic communication.

The setting of boundaries

Notwithstanding the importance of fostering a patient-friendly atmosphere through quality-enhanced communication, maintaining appropriate clinician–patient boundaries is also a necessity. Generally speaking, existing and appropriate boundaries are implicitly understood and entrenched, and need not be addressed. Although the dentist may make a conscious effort to hold his/her emotions in check and allow for free-flowing communication, an excessive expression of emotion is deemed inappropriate. In other words, if a patient's anger takes on vituperative tones, or if a patient's anxiety takes on a diffuse and overwhelming quality, or if a patient places excessive or improper demands on the dentist, a referral to a different practitioner may be in order. When patients exhibit diagnosable anxiety-related disorders, mood disorders, or somatoform disorders, it is incumbent on the dentist to contemplate a referral or to resolve to engage in a collaborative alliance with a mental health professional.

At times, it might be necessary to set limits on a patient's behavior by clarifying office procedures/policies, emphasizing the necessity for respecting the functions of office staff, or explaining the nature of phone interactions. Such discussions should be undertaken with a minimum of intensity and in respectful tones. Termination of service is mentioned only if the efforts alluded to prove fruitless.

In an earlier section of this article, the BATHE approach was introduced as a tool that could serve to minimize difficulties that might arise in clinician–patient encounters, and is worthy of review.

Stress management techniques for quality-of-life enhancement

Unchecked long-term stress can lead to significant physical and emotional consequences. Goldstein and McEwen [56] emphasize that short- and long-term stress elicit different types of physical responses. The brain's short-term response to stress is referred to as allostasis and can actually be protective. The stress hormone, cortisol, and other stress-related responses stimulate the cardiovascular system, the memory processes, and the immune system. Nonetheless, the long-term consequence of stress, referred to as allostatic load, have an antithetic effect because long-term stress will ultimately suppress immune system functioning and compromise memory processes. However, stress management measures, such as progressive relaxation training and physical exercise, and socially supportive endeavors can minimize allostatic load. Numerous studies highlight the benefits of stress management interventions and the prevention and control of hypertension. In a meta-analysis spanning 30 years of research, with a focus on the health-inducing and restorative effects of stress management techniques such as cognitive-behavioral interventions, behavioral relaxation procedures, meditation, and biofeedback, Spence and colleagues [57] were able to show that such interventions lead to consistent reductions in blood pressure readings. They emphasize that although no direct evidence exists that stress management interventions can prevent hypertension, a preponderance of evidence suggests that the implementation of stress management can effectively lower the blood pressure of hypertensives. The most efficacious approach appears to be the use of a multicomponent strategy in applying stress management techniques (eg, combining cognitive reframing instructions with PMR procedures).

Denollet [26] described the type D personality as a refinement of the types A and C personality subtype concepts. Using a 14-item questionnaire, he was able to identify individuals who were approximately four times more likely than others to experience fatal heart attacks or death 6 to 9 months subsequent to coronary artery surgery. Individuals with a type D personality makeup tend to suppress their negative emotions, remain in a state of chronic stress, persist in pessimistic mental frames following their surgeries, and keep the lethal factor, intense distress, active.

Benson and Stuart [58] and other researchers emphasize the need for the individual to recognize the daily stressors by which he/she is affected. Accordingly, Benson and Stuart categorize symptoms exhibited by individuals that are suggestive of a stress response as physical, behavioral, emotional, or cognitive in nature. Examples of physical manifestations of stress include neck and shoulder muscle tension (which yield higher microvoltage readings on electromyogram biofeedback apparatus); lower back pain; a general sense of fatigue; tachycardia; tremors; profuse sweating; gastric distress; restlessness; tinnitus; bruxism; and nausea. Examples of behavioral symptoms include avoidance or procrastination in routines; fidgeting; fist clenching; excessive smoking or overeating; social withdrawal; and frequent complaining. Examples of emotional responses include hyperexcitability or irritability; displays of explosive temper; depression; pervasive diffuse anxiety or subjective sensations of tension and pressure; expressed feelings of isolation; and anhedonia. Examples of cognitive indicators include frequent worrisome thoughts; poor concentration; indecisiveness; poor memory; and exaggerated perception of the difficulties one faces.

Benson [59] advocates using the techniques of deep breathing and PMR, in addition to engaging in enjoyable diversions, to achieve stress reduction. The cognitive technique referred to as cognitive restructuring is an approach that aims to negate automatic or conditioned negative thoughts through mentally reframing such percepts, ideally leading to more rational and less stressful cognitions [60].

The final segment of this article is devoted to a brief and selective overview of available stress management tools and the interventions designed to assist the dentist in achieving an improved quality of life.

Cognitive restructuring

In this cognitive technique, the individual reframes or amends the ways in which he/she thinks about, or how he/she perceives, the problematic or stressful situation or challenge. If one is able to "rewrite" or reframe one's inner thoughts and reactions to an event, one's perception of the event will then be revised so that the same perceived event is viewed as a less threatening encounter. Cognitive behaviorists, such as Albert Ellis [61], have determined that such inner negative percepts and corresponding reactions stem from the individual's tendency to "awfulize" or to engage in "catastrophic-like" thinking. Often, such negative cognitions operate in concert with negative self-percepts. If one is able to learn, through brief cognitive behavioral therapy, how to minimize, or even eradicate, self-castigations and irrational perceptions, one will most certainly have acquired an effective stress management technique.

Progressive muscle relaxation

The PMR technique provides a noticeable sense of relaxation, even after the first application, and the effect is generally achieved after a 15- to 30-minute exercise. The individual is instructed (or self-instructs) to tense and relax muscle groups systematically throughout the body and to be sensitive to the relaxed sensations the experiencc induces. Excellent sources detailing the mechanics of PMR, and discussions describing the benefits that accrue to the individual, are provided in the References section of this article [62–65], on select Web sites devoted to stress management (http://www.guidetopsychology.com/stress.htm), and in the project *Stress Management from Mind Tools* (http://www.mindtools.com/smpage.html).

Guided imagery

The guided imagery technique is often effectively combined with the PMR procedure. Once the individual has undergone relaxation induction, he/she navigates through positive mental imagery with the guidance of the therapist, which allows the individual to achieve an even deeper, more satisfying form of relaxation. Typically, the therapist helps the patient conjure up a personally relaxing scene (foreknowledge of such a scene is elicited through prior discussion). Examples of positive imagery include contemplating or conjuring up relaxing scenes of nature, such as resting beside a lake with a backdrop of a mountain view. The net effect is the achievement of deep relaxation that arrives naturally.

Diaphragmatic breathing

Kabat-Zinn [63] describes the dynamics of the diaphragmatic breathing technique. The abdomen is relaxed, and inhalation proceeds with an accompanying expansion of the abdomen. As the diaphragm expands, the lungs take in more air, which is subsequently expelled during expiration. This breathing becomes deeper and slower and tends to dissipate muscular tension centered in the area of the diaphragm. Proper diaphragmatic breathing leads to a natural relaxation response, which effectively reduces sensations of tension. Williams and Steele [66] assert that when diaphragmatic breathing, PMR, and guided imagery are all undertaken in combination, a profound sense of relaxation is bound to ensue. When the negative emotions of anger, anxiety, hyperirritability, or sympathetic nervous arousal have risen to an uncomfortable degree, diaphragmatic breathing, separately applied or in combination with other relaxation techniques, should be considered.

Mindfulness meditation or insight meditation

The mindfulness meditation or insight meditation approach offers an alternative to the relaxation techniques described earlier [66]. This method requires the individual to attend to or to concentrate fully on a single experience that is occurring at that precise moment. It can be practiced anywhere, and at all times. One can decide to focus on one's breathing, on a specific emotion or thought, or even on the experience of tasting a food item. With concentrated focus, one's awareness and insights are enhanced. By becoming more mindful, one can become more cognizant of what might be personally troublesome. The next step is to let go of self-sabotaging cognitions and to be more mindful of the impact we have on others. Fifteen minutes is generally required to practice mindfulness. Other approaches, such as exercise workouts, yoga, tai chi, and Qi Gong, can also reduce stress.

As we effectively manage the stress we experience in our lives, we become aware that our perceptions, in general, become more rational, and the intensity of our emotions become more appropriate.

Acknowledgments

The author wishes to acknowledge the invaluable assistance of Mr. Joseph Krasner in providing key and seminal research articles germane to the issues addressed in the article. In addition, special thanks is given to Ms. Tanisha Tate for her devotion and assistance in the preparation of this article.

References

[1] Rada RE, Johnson-Leong C. Stress, burnout, anxiety and depression among dentists. J Am Dent Assoc 2004;135:788–94.

[2] Butcher JN, Mineka S, Hooley JM. Abnormal psychology. 12th edition. Boston: Pearson-Allyn Bacon; 2004. p. 140.

[3] Neufeld RW. Coping with stress, coping without stress, and stress with coping; in interconstruct redundancies. Stress Med 1990;6:117–25.
[4] Selye H. Stress in health and disease. Woburn (MA): Butterworth; 1976.
[5] Selye H. The stress of life. 2nd edition. New York: McGraw-Hill; 1976.
[6] Festinger L. A theory of cognitive dissonance. Stanford (CA): Stanford University Press; 1957.
[7] Cannon WB. Bodily changes in pain, hunger, fear and rage. New York: Appleton; 1929.
[8] Erickson K, Drevets W, Schulkin J. Glucocorticoid regulation of diverse cognitive functions in normal and pathological emotional states. Neurosci Biobehav Rev 2003; 27:233–46.
[9] Korte SM. Corticosteroids in relation to fear, anxiety and psychopathology. Neurosci Biobehav Rev 2001;25:117–42.
[10] Stanford SC, Salmon P. Stress: from synapse to syndrome. London: Academic Press; 1993.
[11] Cohen S, Tyrrell DAJ, Smith AP. Psychological stress and susceptibility to the common cold. N Engl J Med 1991;325:606–12.
[12] Adler J. Stress. Newsweek June 14, 1999;58–63.
[13] Dougall AL, Baum A. Stress, health, and illness. In: Baum A, Revenson A, Singer JE, editors. Handbook of health psychology. Mahwah (NJ): Erlbuam; 2001. p. 339–48.
[14] Sternberg EM. The balance within: the science connecting health and emotion. New York: Freeman; 2000.
[15] Kiecolt-Glaser JK, Speicher CE, Holliday JE, et al. Stress and the transformation of lymphocytes in Epstein-Barr virus. J Behav Med 1984;7:1–12.
[16] Salovey P, Rothman AJ, Detweiler JB, et al. Emotional states and physical health. Am Psychol 2000;55:110–21.
[17] Kiecolt-Glaser JK, Page GG, Marucha PT, et al. Psychological influences on surgical recovery. Am Psychol 1998;53:1209–18.
[18] Bodner S. Psychologic considerations in the management of oral surgical patients [In: Dym H, et al, editors]. Oral Maxillofac Surg Clin North Am 2006;18(1):59–72.
[19] Lewinsohn PM, Joiner TE, Rohde P. Evaluation of cognitive diathesis-stress models in predicting major depressive disorder in adolescents. J Abnorm Psychol 2001;110:203–15.
[20] Ormel J, Oldehinkel, Bilman EI. The interplay and the etiological continuity of neuroticism, difficulties, and life events in the etiology of major and subsyndromal, first and recurrent depressive episodes in later life. Am J Psychiatry 2001;158:885–91.
[21] Schwartz BS, Stewart WF, Simon D, et al. Epidemiology of tension-type headache. JAMA 1998;279:381–3.
[22] Sorbi MJ, Maasen GA, Spierings ECH. A time series analysis of daily hassles and mood changes in the 3 days before the migraine attack. Behav Med 1996;22:103–13.
[23] Miller SD, Blackburn T, Scholes G, et al. Optical differences in multiple personality disorder: a second look. J Nerv Ment Dis 1991;179:132–5.
[24] Donker FJS. Cardiac rehabilitation: a review of current developments. Clin Psychol Rev 2000;20:923–43.
[25] Bloom LJ. Psychology and cardiology: collaboration in coronary treatment and prevention. Prof Psychol 1979;10:485–90.
[26] Denollet J. Standard assessments of negative affectivity, social inhibition, and TYPE D personality. Psychosom Med 2005;67(1):89–97.
[27] Krantz DS, Contrada RJ, Hills DR, et al. Enviornmental stress and biobehavioral antecedents of coronary heart disease. J Consult Clin Psychol 1988;56:333–41.
[28] Jorgensen RS, Johnson BT, Kolodenez ME, et al. Elevated blood pressure and personality: a meta-analytic review. Psychol Bull 1996;120:293–320.
[29] Overmier JB, Murison R. Animal models reveal the "psych" in the psychosomatics of peptic ulcers. Curr Dir Psychol Sci 1997;6:180–4.
[30] O'Leary A, Savard J, Miller SM. Psychoimmunology: elucidating the process. Curr Opin Psychiatry 1996;9:427–32.

[31] Sklar LS, Anisman H. Stress and cancer. Psychol Bull 1981;89:369–406.
[32] Ben-Eliyahu S, Shakhar G, Page GG, et al. Suppression of NK cell activity and the resistance to metastasis by stress: a role of adrenal-catecholamines and beta-adrenoceptors. Neuroimmunomodulation 2000;8:154–64.
[33] Quan N, Avitsur R, Stark JL, et al. Social stress increases the susceptibility to endotoxic shock. J Neuroimmunol 2001;115:36–45.
[34] Segerstrom SC, Miller GE. Psychological stress and the human immune system: a meta-analytic study of 30 years of inquiry. Psychol Bull 2004;130:601–30.
[35] Rao JK, Weinberger M, Kroenke K. Visit-specific expectations and patient-centered outcomes. Arch Fam Med 2000;9:1148–55.
[36] Elder N, Ricer R, Tobias B. How respected family physicians manage difficult patient encounters. American Board of Family Medicine 2006;19(6):533–41.
[37] Lin EH, Katon W, Von Korff M, et al. Frustrating patients: physician and patient perspectives among distressed high users of medical services. Journal of General Internal Medicine 1991;6:241–6.
[38] Hahn SR, Kroenke K, Spitzer RL, et al. The difficult patient: prevalence, psychopathology and functional impairment. J Gen Intern Med 1996;11:1–8.
[39] Jackson JL, Kroenke K. Difficult patient encounters in the ambulatory clinic: clinical predictors and outcomes. Arch Intern Med 1999;159:1069–75.
[40] Bodner S. Psychologic aspects of chronic pain. In: Dym H, editor. Oral and maxillofacial surgery clinics of North America: diagnosis and management of facial pain. Philadelphia: Elsevier/Saunders; 2000. p. 181–202.
[41] Steinmetz D, Tabenkin H. The difficult patient as perceived by family physicians. Fam Pract 2001;18:495–500.
[42] McCullough J, Ramesar S, Peterson H. Psychotherapy in primary care: the BATHE technique. Am Fam Physician 1998;57:2131–4.
[43] Essary A, Symington SL. How to make the 'difficult' patient encounter less difficult. JAAPA 2005;18(5):49–54.
[44] Fernandez E, Turk DC. The scope and significance of anger in the experience of chronic pain. Pain 1995;61:161–75.
[45] Burns JW, Johnson BJ, Devine J, et al. Anger management style and the prediction of treatment outcome among male and female chronic pain patients. Behav Res Ther 1998;36: 1051–62.
[46] Ploghaus A, Tracey I, Gati JS, et al. Dissociating pain from its anticipation in the human brain. Science 1999;284:1979–82.
[47] McCracken LM, Gross RT. The Pain Anxiety Symptons Scale (PASS) and the assessment of emotional responses to pain. In: Vandecreeek L, et al, editors. Innovations in clinical practice: a sourcebook. Sarasota (FL): Professional Resource Press; 1995. p. 309–21.
[48] McCraken LM, Zayfert C, Gross RT. The Pain Anxiety Symptoms Scale: development and validation of a scale to measure fear of pain. Pain 1992;50:67–73.
[49] Johnston M, Vogele C. Benefits of psychological preparation for surgery: a meta-analysis. Ann Behav Med 1993;15:245–56.
[50] Haas LJ, Leiser JP, MaGill MK, et al. Management of the difficult patient. Am Fam Physician 2005;72(10):2063–7.
[51] US Department of Health and Human Services-Substance Abuse and Mental Health Services Administration Center for Substance Abuse Treatment. Quick guide for clinicians, based on tip 26: substance abuse among older adults. Washington, DC: Department of Health and Human Services; 2001. p. 26 DHHS publication no. (SMA) 01-3585.
[52] Platt FW, Gordon GH. Field guide to the difficult patient interview. Philadelphia: Lippincott Williams and Wilkins; 2004.
[53] White MK, Keller VF. Difficult clinician-patient relationships. Journal of Clinical Outcome Management 1998;5(5):32–6.

[54] McDevitt TM, Omrod JE. Child development: educating and working with children and adolescents. 2nd edition. Upper Saddle River (NJ): Pearson-Merrill Prentice Hall; 2004. p. 378.
[55] Epstein RM. The science of patient-centered care. J Fam Pract 2000;49:805–7.
[56] Goldstein DS, McEwen B. Allostasis, homeostats and the nature of stress. Stress 2002;5(1): 55–98.
[57] Spence DJ, Barnett PA, Linden W, et al. Recommendations on stress management. Can Med Assoc J 1999;160(9):546–50.
[58] Benson H, Stuart EM. The wellness book. New York: Birch Lane Press; 1993.
[59] Benson H. Stress management: techniques for preventing and easing stress. Boston: Harvard Health Publications; 2006.
[60] Sarason IG, Sarason BR. Abnormal psychology: the problem of maladaptive behavior. 9th edition. Upper Saddle River (NJ): Prentice Hall; 1999.
[61] Ellis A. Humanistic psychotherapy: the rational emotive approach. New York: Julian Press; 1973.
[62] Williams RW, Williams V. Anger kills. New York: Harper Collins; 1993.
[63] Kabat-Zinn J. Full catastrophe living. New York: Dell; 1990.
[64] Benson H. The relaxation response. New York: Harpertorch; 2000.
[65] Elkin A. Stress management for dummies. New York: Wiley; 1999.
[66] Williams MA, Steele MG. Assessment and treatment of psychosocial issues with cardiac patients. In: Vandecreek L, Allen JB, editors. Innovations in clinical practice: focus on health and wellness. Sarasota (FL): Professional Resource Press; 2005. p. 87–104.

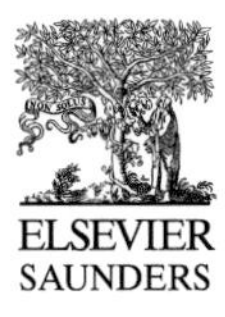

ELSEVIER
SAUNDERS

Dent Clin N Am 52 (2008) 605–608

THE DENTAL CLINICS OF NORTH AMERICA

Preparing the Dental Office for Medical Emergencies

Harry Dym, DDS[a,b,c,*]

[a]*Department of Dentistry and Oral Maxillofacial Surgery, The Brooklyn Hospital Center, 121 Dekalb Avenue, Brooklyn, NY 11201, USA*
[b]*Woodhull Hospital, Brooklyn, NY, USA*
[c]*Department of Oral and Maxillofacial Surgery, Columbia University College of Dental Medicine, New York, NY, USA*

When planning to open a private office that is patient oriented, employee friendly, and doctor centered, knowledge in many nonclinical areas such as patient billing, infection control, accounting, and so forth is, of course, mandatory. However, an area that is most critical but sometimes overlooked by dentists when establishing new offices is preparation for the management of office medical emergencies. Although such office medical emergencies are infrequent, the dentist will often be held legally responsible for any untoward outcome allegedly resulting from causation or mismanagement of those medical emergencies. With the elderly population growing, the number of patients who are on multiple medications for underlying medical conditions will certainly be increasing.

This article does not focus on the diagnosis and management of specific medical and dental emergencies, or on a detailed pharmacologic discussion of the drugs used, but rather, on the policies, equipment, and personnel needed to prepare for dealing with emergencies, should they occur. No discussion of techniques or the underlying physiology is discussed because this information is readily available elsewhere [1,2].

Office equipment

Dental offices should be prepared to provide basic airway management, which includes the ability to administer 100% oxygen through a portable O_2 source. One "E" oxygen tank, when full, will last approximately 60

* Department of Dentistry and Oral Maxillofacial Surgery, The Brooklyn Hospital Center, 121 Dekalb Avenue, Brooklyn, NY 11201.
E-mail address: hdymdds@yahoo.com

0011-8532/08/$ - see front matter
doi:10.1016/j.cden.2008.02.010

minutes when given at a 10 L per minute flow rate. The dentist must frequently check to ascertain the O_2 tank status, even if two tanks are available for backup. Oxygen can be delivered by way of a nasal cannula, face mask, or face mask with reservoir. It is the author's opinion that all offices should have an Ambu bag and a full face mask, merely to allow the dentist to provide positive pressure ventilation should the need rise. A nasal and oral airway should also be part of most dentists' airway management kit.

Stethoscope and sphygmomanometer (with child- and adult-size cuffs) and an assortment of syringes and needles should also be considered as part of the dental office's basic emergency equipment. The one device that has now become ubiquitous in its presence in almost all public places is the automatic external defibrillator (AED). The survival rate in cardiac arrests approaches 30% if early defibrillation is administered, accompanied by advance cardiac life support. The AED also eliminates the need for training in rhythm recognition but it does require the dentist and key staff to be trained in its use by participating in the American Heart Association's basic cardiopulmonary resuscitation course. See Box 1.

Emergency drugs

General dentists and dental specialists should develop an emergency box that is dedicated to emergencies and stocked with the following key basic resuscitation drugs. Those offices providing intravenous sedation will certainly have more comprehensive emergency drugs available.

Aromatic ammonia: Syncope is the most common medical emergency in the dental office. Vaporable aromatic ammonia is available and, when

Box 1. Basic emergency equipment

Tourniquets
Syringes
Ambu bag
Oropharyngeal and nasopharyngeal airways
Normal saline 0.9%, 1000-mL bags
18-and 20-gauge angiocatheters
Yankauer suction tip
Portable oxygen system (E cylinder size)
Stethoscope
Sphygmomanometer (child and adult sizes)
EKG/defibrillator (AED)
Sterile water for injection

cracked or crushed, it releases a noxious odor that stimulates the respiratory and vasomotor centers of the medulla. When combined with placing the patient in a Trendelenburg's position and providing supplemental oxygen, most patients will return to consciousness.

Aspirin: The American Heart Association recommends that patients experiencing an acute myocardial infarction chew an aspirin. Chewing a buffered aspirin (325 mg) for 30 seconds and then swallowing it with water is thought to have a rapid and sustained effect.

Nitroglycerine: Nitroglycerine is recommended for relief of angina in patients who have a past history, and for those with a new onset of angina with a suspected myocardial infarction. Nitroglycerin is available as a 0.4-mg metered aerosol. The spray does not require special storage and has a 3-year shelf life; the tablet form requires special storage in light-resistant containers and loses its potency in 12 weeks. Administration of this drug is safe, with headaches, dizziness, and flushing as possible side effects.

Inhaled $beta_2$-agonists: Bronchodilators are the main drug groups used for the treatment of wheezing and bronchospasm. Selective $beta_2$-agonists are the preferred drugs because they minimize the side effects, including tachycardia, hypertension, angina, restlessness, and flushing. Albuterol is the preferred choice because it is the most selective of the $beta_2$-agonists and it comes in a metered dose inhaler.

Epinephrine: Epinephrine is a sympathomimetic drug that acts on alpha adrenergic and beta adrenergic receptors with primary effects being bronchodilation, vasoconstriction, and increased rate and force of cardiac contraction, along with stabilization of mast cells (involved in severe allergic reactions.) See Box 2.

Hypoglycemic agent (D50W): The purpose of oral hypoglycemic agents is to increase blood glucose levels in patients who are conscious and hypoglycemic. All offices should store a simple sugar source such as fruit juices. If the patient cannot swallow, dextrose 50% in water (D50W) should be used by way of any intravenous route.

Box 2. Basic drug emergency kit

Epinephrine 1mg/mL (1:1000 dilution)
D50W 50 mL ampule 0.5g/mL
Oxygen
Nitroglycerin tablets or spray 0.4 mg per tablet
Albuterol; metered inhaler
Hydrocortisone 300 mg ampule
Spirits of ammonia (vaporable)

Staff and office preparation

The dentist should develop a protocol and policy for his/her staff to follow when a medical emergency arises. The dentist and key staff should be certified in basic life support and trained as first responders. The front office should have the phone numbers of the area's local ambulance or emergency medical service, local emergency department, and an adjacent internist or oral and maxillofacial surgeon in the same building. A code word should be established in the office to inform the staff of an ongoing emergency so that staff can coordinate the proper emergency response.

The emergency kit should be updated regularly and, along with oxygen, should be placed in an area that is readily accessible.

Mock emergencies should be performed regularly so that the staff will respond appropriately should the need arise.

Finally, dental offices should develop "cheat sheets" (these are also available for purchase), cards that list the type of emergency occurring, with the appropriate actions to be taken by the doctor and staff.

References

[1] Dym H. Stocking the oral surgery office emergency cart. In: Ogle OE, editor. Pharmacology, oral and maxillofacial surgery clinics of North America, vol. 13. Philadelphia: Saunders; 2001.

[2] Saef SN, Bennett JD. Basic principles and resuscitation. In: Bennett JD, Rosenberg MB, editors. Medical emergencies in dentistry. Saunders; 2002.

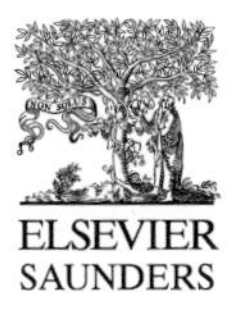

ELSEVIER
SAUNDERS

THE DENTAL CLINICS OF NORTH AMERICA

Dent Clin N Am 52 (2008) 609–628

Infection Control in the Dental Office

Mark V. Thomas, DMD[a,*], Glena Jarboe[b], Robert Q. Frazer, DDS[c]

[a]*Division of Periodontology, University of Kentucky, College of Dentistry, 800 Rose Street, Lexington, KY 40536-0297, USA*
[b]*University of Kentucky, College of Dentistry, 800 Rose Street, Room M 128, Lexington, KY 40536-0297, USA*
[c]*Division of Prosthodontics, University of Kentucky, College of Dentistry, 800 Rose Street, Lexington, KY 40536-0297, USA*

Dental health care personnel (DHCP) work in close proximity to their patients. DHCP perform procedures which may induce their patients to cough. Their field of surgery is awash in saliva, which is usually contaminated with blood. Many dental procedures produce aerosolized droplet nuclei, which may linger in the atmosphere for hours. Obviously, the risk of disease transmission is an inherent part of dental practice. The good news is that dental care can be provided with a high degree of safety for the patient and therapist, provided that the tenets of modern infection control are adhered to. One of the most comprehensive sources of information regarding infection control practices in the dental setting is available from the Centers for Disease Control and Prevention [1].

The office safety and infection control (SIC) program provides a framework in which dental treatment can be rendered safely and effectively. The ultimate legal responsibility for implementing such a program resides with the owner of the practice, but the plan requires the full cooperation of the entire staff.

An infection control (IC) plan–that is part of a larger safety plan–has as its goal the protection of patients and health care workers. The plan must provide for:

- creation of IC protocols designed to safeguard the health and safety of both patients and staff;
- ongoing training;
- surveillance of infection control hazards and exposures;

* Corresponding author.
E-mail address: mvthom0@uky.edu (M.V. Thomas).

0011-8532/08/$ - see front matter
doi:10.1016/j.cden.2008.02.002
dental.theclinics.com

- ongoing quality assurance and continuous improvement;
- regulatory compliance.

It may be helpful to designate a staff member as the SIC officer who is responsible for plan implementation, staff training, and quality assurance.

Standard precautions

Transmission of bloodborne pathogens can normally be prevented through the use of standard precautions. The Centers for Disease Control (CDC) defines standard precautions as "any standard of care designed to protect health care personnel and patients from pathogens that can be spread by blood or any other bodily fluid, excretion, or secretion." The term "standard precautions" replaces the term "universal precautions." Standard precautions apply to contact with blood, bodily fluids (except sweat), intact mucous membranes, and non-intact skin. These precautions are normally sufficient to prevent the transmission of infectious agents in the dental setting.

Records maintenance and security

Employers must create and maintain confidential health records for all employees. Such information must be maintained in secure files for the duration of employment plus 30 years [2]. These records must contain immunization records, occupational exposures to bloodborne pathogens (BBP), injuries, and medical work restrictions. It is also necessary to keep records of training, including information like dates, presenters, and topics. Training records should be kept for at least 3 years [2].

Infection control training

Who must be trained?

Mandatory infection control training is needed by any staff members who are at risk of exposure to bloodborne pathogens. This would include all clinical staff, including laboratory technicians, but may also include administrative personnel who have contact with patients and handle charts (which may be contaminated). For each individual practice, practice owners are legally obligated to assess the potential risk inherent in each position and train staff accordingly. Staff members who are to be included in such training will hereafter be referred to as "clinical staff" regardless of the exact nature of their duties.

Volunteers and observers

It is not uncommon for volunteers and observers to be present in the clinical environment. While this is more common in institutions such as dental schools, it is also common in dental practices, especially those in which dental or hygiene students must rotate. At our institution, such individuals receive abbreviated training in the Health Insurance Portability and Accountability Act of 1996 (HIPAA) and IC. Such individuals may be injured during their observational experience. If such individuals are present in the practice, an appropriate policy should be developed regarding mandatory training, hepatitis B immunization, and postexposure protocol should an injury occur. Appropriate legal counsel should be sought in developing these guidelines.

When should such training be taken?

All clinical staff must receive mandatory training in safety and infection control. All training must be documented in an employee training record. Training must be received at the time of initial assignment, or whenever there are changes in procedure or clinical responsibilities. Training should be conducted annually thereafter. Training sessions should be held during working hours. It may be convenient to review IC issues at monthly staff meetings on an ongoing basis. If this is done, a formal record of the training should be kept for all attendees.

What topics must be covered?

At a minimum, training should cover: the Occupational Safety and Health Administration (OSHA) Standard; bloodborne diseases (especially hepatitis B [including information on immunization], hepatitis C, and HIV/AIDS); the office-specific exposure control plan; the use and care of personal protective equipment (PPE); postexposure protocol; and hazard communication (eg, biohazard symbols).

Resources

Many videos and instructional materials are available for training. However, the training must be specific and appropriate to the individual office. Also, employees must be given the opportunity to ask questions. The written IC plan must also be specific to the individual office. It is acceptable, however, to use a generic IC video if it is followed by an office-specific training session. Following the initial training session(s), there should be an annual IC update.

General information on infection control is available from a number of sources. Chief among these are the latest guidelines from the Centers for Disease Control and Prevention (ie, *Guidelines for Infection Control in Dental Healthcare Settings – 2003*) [1]. Information is also available from OSHA (www.osha.gov), the National Institute for Occupational Health (NIOSH; www.cdc.gov/niosh/), the American Dental Association (ADA; http://www.ada.org/), the Organization for Safety and Asepsis Procedures

(OSAP; http://www.osap.org/), and the Association for Professionals in Infection Control and Epidemiology (APIC; http://www.apic.org). The *Regulatory Compliance Manual* is available from the ADA and is a good source of general information [3].

Nature of the threat

Theoretically, almost any infectious disease could be transmitted in the dental setting, but there are a few diseases that are of special importance. These significant diseases include hepatitis B, hepatitis C, HIV, and tuberculosis. An exposure is said to exist when an individual has possibly come in contact with such pathogens. An accidental needlestick is an example of a percutaneous exposure. Other exposures can occur when a piece of calculus lands in an assistant's eye or when airborne infections are spread by aerosols generated by a dental handpiece or by a patient's sneeze or cough.

Standard precautions are effective in breaking the chain of infection, since transmission of the hepatitis B virus is rare in cases where proper IC protocols are followed. Even when an exposure occurs, infection is not inevitable. The risk of infection following exposure is determined by a number of factors, including inoculum size (ie, how big a dose of organisms the person is exposed to), the method of exposure (material splashed in the eye versus needlestick), and the susceptibility of the host.

Inoculum size is an important concern in determining the risk of infection. Hollow needles, which can carry a larger number of pathogens due to the hollow channel or lumen within the needle, are much more effective in transmitting infection than solid instruments such as suture needles. The rate of infection following needlestick is also dependent upon the pathogen. For example, the rate of infection following a needlestick (ie, percutaneous) injury is greater for cases of hepatitis B virus (6%–30%) than for hepatitis C virus (0%–7%) or HIV (0.3%) [1,4].

Viral hepatitis

Hepatitis is a generic term that means inflammation of the liver. Hepatitis can be caused by viral and bacterial infections, by other parasites, or by exposure to chemicals and drugs (such as alcohol). Viral hepatitis is caused by any of a number of viruses [5]. Three types of viral hepatitis are especially important in the dental setting.

Hepatitis B

Hepatitis B is caused by the hepatitis B virus (HBV) [6,7]. Hepatitis B is the bloodborne pathogen most likely to be encountered in the dental workplace. HBV is also persistent. The viral particles may remain infectious for a week in dried blood at room temperature. In dentistry, the most common route of transmission from patient to DHCP is from a percutaneous exposure via needlestick or a similar event. For this reason, it is the target organism for infection control measures. If IC measures are effective in preventing the transmission of hepatitis B, they will probably be effective in preventing the transmission of most other bloodborne diseases.

There are an estimated 200 to 300 million carriers of HBV worldwide, with over 1 million Americans chronically infected. Certain high-risk populations have been identified, such as health care workers, intravenous drug users, female prostitutes, male homosexuals, and immigrants from certain regions having a high prevalence of HBV (eg, Asia, Africa, the Middle East, Haiti). However, it is important to note that anyone can be a carrier of HBV. Approximately 10% of those with primary HBV infection eventually become carriers. Although several markers (antigens) are characteristic of HBV, the one most often used to determine infectivity in asymptomatic carriers is the hepatitis B surface antigen. HBV carriers are at greatly increased risk for hepatocellular carcinoma, cirrhosis, and transmission to family members.

The symptoms of the initial HBV infection are often mild, and the infected individual may mistake them for influenza. Most individuals with HBV do not experience jaundice during the initial infection. HBV causes over 4000 deaths per year in the United States. Fortunately, the incidence of HBV is declining due to the combined effects of improved IC practices, better education, and the availability of an effective vaccine.

The availability and wide use of the HBV vaccine has greatly reduced the number of infected health care workers; it is a public health success story. All health care workers should be vaccinated against hepatitis B. Currently available forms of the vaccine are 98%–99% effective. Three injections are required in the series. All DHCP should be immunized against HBV within 10 days of their first contact with patients. Individuals may see patients during the period (normally 2–6 months) that it takes to complete the immunization series. Any DHCP who do not wish to be immunized must sign a form of declination that should be kept in the employee's file. An example of such a letter is found in the appendix. Employers are responsible for offering this immunization to their patients free of charge. Upon hiring new clinical DHCP, an employer may wish to see evidence of immunization although this is not mandated by OSHA.

Hepatitis C

Hepatitis C virus (HCV) is the most common cause of so-called "non-A, non-B hepatitis [7–11]." Eighty percent of HCV infections result in a chronic carrier state, which contributes to the importance of this agent. It is estimated that there are almost 4 million infected persons in the United States, including over 2 million infectious carriers. Risk factors for HCV include exposure to blood and body fluids (eg, needlesticks, sharing needles) and multiple sex partners. In many cases, no risk factor can be identified. No effective vaccine exists for hepatitis C.

Hepatitis D

Hepatitis D is unique because the virus can only replicate in the presence of the hepatitis B virus [1,7]. Patients infected with both HBV and the hepatitis D virus (HDV) sometimes have a particularly severe form of hepatitis known as fulminant hepatitis. Because HDV requires coinfection with HBV, it is likely that vaccination against HBV will also provide protection against HDV.

HIV

In 1981, the CDC published the first reports of unusual opportunistic infections in homosexual men in Los Angeles [12,13]. These men were diagnosed with *Pneumocystis carinii* pneumonia (PCP), an infection not usually seen in healthy young adults. This brief report signaled the beginning of the AIDS epidemic, a public health event that transformed health care and focused increased attention on infection control.

Although the AIDS epidemic focused increased attention on IC in the dental setting, the danger of transmission in this setting is apparently low. According to the CDC, as of December 2001 there were no reports of transmission of HIV to DHCP as a result of workplace exposures. There is one report of HIV transmission from a dentist to several patients, but the mode of transmission has never been ascertained and this appears to be a highly unusual, isolated case.

In an effort to quantify the risk of transmission from health care worker to patient, the CDC examined over 22,000 patients who were treated by 63 HIV-infected health care providers (including 33 dentists or dental students) and found no additional cases of transmission. It would appear that the risk of transmission in the dental workplace is quite low.

Routes of HIV transmission include contact with contaminated blood, other body fluids, or other potentially infectious material (OPIM). Transmission can occur via sexual contact, needle sharing, and vertical transmission from mother to child. HIV-positive individuals may remain asymptomatic for years. Eventually, however, the immune system fails and the person develops AIDS. The virus is shed in blood and saliva, and low viral levels have been found in oral secretions. There is no cure for AIDS, although new drug regimens, such as highly active antiretroviral therapy, have proven much more effective than older protocols. The new protocols have resulted in greatly increased longevity for AIDS patients.

Tuberculosis

Tuberculosis (TB) is caused by the tubercle bacillus, *Mycobacterium tuberculosis* (Mtb) [14–18]. TB is spread chiefly through extremely small airborne droplet nuclei produced when an infected individual sneezes, coughs, or speaks. These droplet nuclei can remain airborne for hours. However, contact with Mtb is not sufficient to cause active tuberculosis. Many individuals have been exposed to the organism and have developed a latent infection (as indicated by a positive TB skin test), but only about 10% of these individuals will develop active TB during their lifetime. (This proportion is greatly increased in persons infected with HIV.) In many cases, the organism remains in a latent or hidden state. In some cases, these latent tuberculosis infections (LTBI) may be reactivated when immune function deteriorates (eg, due to AIDS or increasing age). TB is the most common cause of death from infectious disease in the world, particularly in parts of the former Soviet Union, Asia and Mexico. Of great concern in these areas is the emergence of multidrug-resistant TB.

Prion diseases

Prion diseases are unique [1,19]. Prions are not bacteria and they are not viruses. In fact, they are infectious proteins that lack a genome. It is difficult to imagine prions as living organisms in the generally accepted sense of that term. The best-known example is the so-called "mad cow disease" (also known as bovine spongiform encephalopathy or BSE). Mad cow disease is an example of a group a diseases known as transmissible spongiform encephalopathies or TSEs. Initially, it was recognized that mad cow disease was similar to a human condition known as Creutzfeldt-Jakob disease. It appears that consumption of meat tainted with the BSE agent may result in human infection known as variant CJD.

Normal methods of sterilization may not be effective in killing or inactivating prions. These diseases have exceptionally long incubation periods (10–30 years) which greatly complicate the epidemiologic study of the mode of transmission. Some materials used in periodontal and oral surgery use materials are derived from cattle (ie, certain collagen membranes, sutures, xenograft bone graft materials), although there have been no reported instances of contamination from these materials.

Other infections

When discussing disease transmission in the dental setting, the focus is naturally upon those infections with the most serious consequences such as AIDS and HBV. However, more common diseases such as the common cold, influenza, various herpes viruses, and STDs may also be transmitted. Some, such as influenza, may have serious sequelae. The safeguards taken to prevent transmission of HBV, for example, will also reduce the chances for transmission of other, more common pathogens. While usually not life-threatening, diseases such as the common cold and herpetic skin infections may be debilitating and unpleasant for dental health care workers and their families.

Breaking the chain of infection

Infectious diseases spread by direct contact between individuals, via airborne droplets, or by contact with fomites such as contaminated surfaces or instruments. One of the most important routes of transmission in the dental workplace is direct exposure to blood and body fluids (BBF), as well as other potentially infectious material (PIM). Blood is the most important fluid. Blood is usually found in saliva, due to gingival bleeding. Therefore, all saliva is considered a potentially infectious material and must be treated with caution.

A number of strategies are available to reduce the possibility of cross-infection. These include training, workplace restrictions, immunization, the use of personal protective equipment, and safe work practices, including the use of safer instruments, such as retractable needles. All of these elements, plus quality assurance mechanisms, should be included in the infection control plan.

Workplace restrictions and immunizations

Medical work restrictions

The presence of certain medical conditions in DHCP may pose a potential threat to patients. Certain of these illnesses require the DHCP to be excluded from clinical duties. Decisions regarding medical restriction should be based on epidemiologic evidence and CDC recommendations. Selected medical conditions and related work restrictions are shown in Table 1.

This table's information is not exhaustive; other conditions and recommendations may be found in the CDC's *Guidelines for Infection Control in Dental Healthcare Settings* (2003). Of particular interest is the increasing incidence of dermatitis secondary to latex allergy and frequent hand hygiene procedures.

Active tuberculosis: a special case

Depending upon the prevalence of TB in a region, it may be prudent to obtain a baseline tuberculin skin test for all DHCP. Depending upon the region, it may be prudent to test DHCP yearly, so that seroconversion rates can be tracked. All DHCP who come in contact with a suspected or confirmed case of active TB must receive a tuberculin skin test (TST). Patients should be routinely asked about history of and exposure to TB. Symptoms and signs of TB include unexplained weight loss, night sweats, fatigue, malaise, bloody sputum, anorexia, fever, and a productive cough lasting longer

Table 1
CDC recommendations on work restrictions for health care personnel

Disease/condition	Work restriction	Duration of restriction
Conjunctivitis	No patient contact	Until discharge ceases
Diarrhea	No patient contact	Until symptoms resolve
Hepatitis A	No patient contact	Until 7 days after onset of jaundice
Hepatitis B (e antigenemia)	No invasive procedures until counsel from review panel sought	Until HBeAg negative; check for latest CDC, state and local regs
Hepatitis C	No restriction	
Herpes simplex, genital	No restriction	
Herpes simplex, whitlow	No patient contact	Until lesions have healed
Herpes simplex, orofacial	Consider restricting care to immunocompetent patients	
HIV infection	No invasive procedures until counsel from review panel sought	
Measles, active	Exclude from duty	Until 7 days after rash appears
Meningococcal infection	Exclude from duty	Until 24 hours after start of effective therapy
Mumps, active	Exclude from duty	Until 9 days after onset of parotitis
Staph aureus infection, draining skin lesion	No patient contact	Until lesions have resolved
Strep infection, group A	No patient contact	Until 24 hours after therapy begun
Tuberculosis, active	Exclude from duty	Until proved noninfectious
Varicella, active	Exclude from duty	Until all lesions dry and crust
Zoster (shingles)	Cover lesions, restrict from care of immunocompromised patient	Until all lesions dry and crust

From Cetron MS, Marfin AA, Julian KG, et al. Yellow fever vaccine. Recommendations of the Advisory Committee on Immunization Practices (ACIP). MMWR 2003;52(No. RR-17):8–9.

than 3 weeks. Patients presenting with such symptoms and signs should be referred for medical evaluation before treatment is rendered, particularly if the individual has risk factors for TB (eg, HIV/AIDS, from an area in which TB is endemic, close contact with active TB case).

Routine dental treatment of active TB patients is contraindicated. Treatment of such patients must take place in a special facility with appropriate engineering controls for airborne infection isolation. Normal surgical masks do not provide sufficient protection; instead, special respirators are required.

Immunization program

All employees, including temporary and part-time employees, must be offered immunization against hepatitis B. This requires a three-dose vaccine series. All employees with clinical exposure must begin this series within 10 days of employment and can see patients while completing the series [3]. Employees who have previously received the vaccine are exempt from this requirement, as are those who are immune (as determined by antibody assay). This immunization must be provided at no cost to the employee. Since a small percentage of individuals do not respond to the initial vaccine, it is recommended that all employees receiving the vaccine be tested for the presence of antibodies. All DHCP are also strongly urged to receive the following vaccinations: influenza, measles (live-virus), mumps (live-virus), rubella (live-virus), and varicella-zoster (live-virus). More details concerning these recommendations are available from the CDC Web site.

Individuals who refuse the recommended immunizations must sign a formal letter indicating that they have declined the opportunity to be immunized, despite being aware of the health risks that this entails.

Exposure control

Hand hygiene

Hand hygiene is one of the simplest and yet one of the most important infection control measures. All DHCP should develop good hand hygiene habits. One of the earliest proponents of hand hygiene was Ignaz Semmelweiss, a 19th century Austrian physician who noted that there was a higher rate of infection in the patients attended by physicians as compared with patients who were treated by midwives. Semmelweiss observed that physicians often came to the ward immediately after performing autopsies and often did not wash their hands. He speculated that the subsequent infections in the postpartum women were due to "cadaveric material" from the physicians' hands. This was a remarkably intuitive insight, considering that the germ theory of disease had not yet been established. Semmelweiss conducted a study in which he required physicians on his service to wash their hands in chlorinated lime solution before they treated patients. This dramatically reduced the rate of infection although many of his colleagues were still skeptical.

For general patient care, hands should be washed with an antimicrobial soap such as 4% chlorhexidine (CHX) when visibly soiled. If the hands are not soiled, an alcohol-based hand rub (AHR) may be used instead. Studies indicate that AHRs are very effective and may be less irritating than some antiseptic soaps. Before performing surgical procedures, hands should be thoroughly scrubbed for 2–6 minutes with CHX or some similar antiseptic soap.

Hand lotions can be used to prevent dryness, but they should be compatible with the gloves. Some emollients in lotions can adversely affect glove integrity. Fingernails should be neatly trimmed and no longer than ¼ ″ long. Artificial nails should not be worn. It is best not to wear rings with sharp edges and prongs because they may cause tears in the gloves.

Personal protective equipment

Employers are responsible for analyzing the hazards in the workplace and providing appropriate personal protective equipment (PPE). Employers must also take reasonable steps to ensure that personnel are compliant in the use of such equipment and that personnel are trained in its use and limitations. Employees must be retrained when new equipment is introduced or when there are perceived inadequacies in the employees' knowledge of such equipment. Records of such training should be kept to document compliance with this regulation.

Masks, eyewear, face shields

A properly fitted surgical mask and protective eyewear with side shields should be worn during procedures that are likely to cause splashing or splattering of blood. This includes various cleanup duties (eg, cleaning plaster traps and evacuation systems) as well as direct patient care. Masks should be changed between patients or if the mask becomes soiled or wet (a not infrequent occurrence). Face shields may be considered for procedures that involve a great potential for splatter or aerosol generation. The mask should not be touched during the procedure. Patients should also be provided with safety glasses during treatment.

Protective clothing

Protective clothing should be worn during patient care and other duties in which splatter or contact with BBF or OPIM is likely. Gowns should completely cover personal clothing and any skin likely to come in contact with bloodborne pathogens. Gowns should be changed if soiled or wet.

All PPE must be removed when leaving the work area. Soiled gowns should be kept in a special receptacle.

Glove use

The concept of gloving for surgical procedures is credited to the American surgeon, Dr. William Halsted. While at Johns Hopkins University, Halsted suggested that the Goodyear Rubber Company develop a thin glove that could be used during surgery. Gloves must be used when exposure to blood or body fluids is likely. Hands should be washed before donning gloves and after their removal. Gloves should never be washed, as this may adversely affect their integrity. Since the likelihood of breaches in glove integrity increase with increasing duration of the procedure, it may be wise to change gloves during particularly long procedures. Surgeons' gloves should be worn during surgical procedures. There is some evidence to suggest that the use of double gloves may offer some additional protection, but the CDC feels that this is an unresolved issue and has made no recommendations regarding this practice.

Gloves should be selected that fit well. Gloves that are too small may cause hand fatigue and cramps. Many individuals are allergic to latex or powder. Such individuals must be provided with an acceptable latex- or powder-free alternative. Questions regarding the suitability of a particular type of glove or compatibility with lotions should be directed to the manufacturer.

After wearing gloves for a period of time, fluid is collected within the glove. This fluid is laden with skin flora and is known as "glove juice." Glove juice is commonly used to test the efficacy of hand sanitizers and surgical disinfectants. It is important, therefore, to prevent glove juice from contacting instruments that will be used in patient care. This is most likely to happen when changing gloves during a long procedure. It is strongly recommended that the clinician remove the gloves slowly and deliberately, with their hands as far away from the instrument setup as possible.

Latex allergy and dermatitis

Latex allergy and contact dermatitis are often seen in health care workers. Personnel should be alert for signs of dermatitis. These signs include itching, redness, rash, dryness, fissures/cracking, hyperkeratosis, and swelling. In some cases, systemic allergic symptoms may be present; symptoms include sneezing, wheezing, urticaria, and red, watery eyes. Medical consultation should be sought and the employee should be provided a latex-free alternative glove.

Because some of these reactions may be due to powder on the glove, powder-free gloves are preferred. Latex-laden powder particles may become airborne and produce symptoms in susceptible individuals even when they are not actually wearing such gloves. For this reason, it may be desirable to create a latex-free environment in the dental office.

Postexposure protocol

In the event of an exposure such as a needlestick, the DHCP should stop the procedure, gently cleanse the wound, and notify the supervisor. The source patient should be encouraged to be tested for the presence of bloodborne pathogens, although they cannot be forced to do so. Depending on an analysis of the patient's medical status and risk factors for bloodborne disease (eg, parenteral drug abuse), a qualified physician will determine the need for postexposure prophylaxis (PEP). As a result of this assessment, the exposed worker could require a prolonged course of antiretroviral agents or no treatment other than first aid. The latest PEP recommendations can be found on the CDC Web site (www.cdc.gov).

Following exposure, a formal incident analysis should occur as soon as possible to determine what can be done to reduce the risk of recurrence. It would be prudent to keep a log of such exposures and their disposition.

Environmental infection control

Environmental surfaces in the dental treatment area are assumed to be contaminated due to the aerosols generated during dental procedures. These surfaces can be separated into housekeeping surfaces (such as floors) and clinical contact surfaces. Clinical contact surfaces include the handles and switch of the dental light, power switches, and other controls on the dynamic instrument arm that contains the handpieces. Clinical contact surfaces are often touched during treatment, allowing organisms to be transferred from the surface to the patient or DHCP. For this reason, clinical contact surfaces require more thorough disinfection than housekeeping surfaces.

PPE should be worn when performing housekeeping and clean-up duties. At a minimum, PPE should include protective clothing, protective eyewear, and puncture resistant nitrile gloves.

Barriers and surface disinfection

Barriers should be used to protect clinical surfaces that cannot be easily cleaned. Such surfaces include the handles of the operatory light, the bracket tray/arm/handpiece console, and the dental chair. The armrest of the assistant's stool may similarly be covered. If any clinical surface cannot be covered with a barrier, then it must be disinfected using an intermediate-level (ie, tuberculocidal) EPA-registered disinfectant. Visible blood and debris must be removed before disinfection, as organic debris will interfere with the action of the disinfectant. Some equipment manufacturers recommend that surface disinfectants not be used on the upholstered portion of the chair unless the surface is contaminated. If barriers are used to cover such surfaces, further disinfection is not necessary, unless the integrity of the barrier is breached.

Housekeeping surfaces

Floors, walls, and sinks must be cleaned with detergent/water or an EPA-registered hospital disinfectant/detergent on a regular basis. Such surfaces must be cleaned if visibly soiled. Treatment areas should be free of extraneous materials to facilitate cleaning and disinfection. Loose items should be placed in drawers or other storage.

Blood spills

Spills of blood or other grossly contaminated liquid (eg, as might be encountered when cleaning a plaster trap) should be cleaned with an intermediate-level (ie, tuberculocidal) EPA-registered disinfectant.

Laboratory precautions

Dental impressions and prostheses may be contaminated with BBF which will cause them to pose a threat to DHCP and patients. Special precautions must be taken to prevent cross-contamination. Prostheses, orthodontic devices, impressions, and occlusal registrations should be thoroughly cleaned and disinfected with an EPA-registered tuberculocidal disinfectant before being sent to the laboratory (whether in-house or extramural). The manufacturer of the impression material should be contacted to ensure that these agents do not adversely affect the accuracy of the impression. Similarly, prostheses and appliances should be disinfected before delivery to the patient. Contaminated materials sent to an extramural laboratory are subject to OSHA and US Department of Transportation regulations and they may require special handling.

Laboratory equipment and instruments should be heat-sterilized or disinfected between patients. These items include pumice, muslin buff wheels, and other abrasive materials. If ultrasonic cleaners are used to clean prostheses or other items that are to be inserted in the patient's mouth, the prosthesis must first be placed in a sealed, impervious receptacle containing cleaner.

Sterilization and instrument processing

Contaminated instruments must be sterilized between patients. Critical items (ie, those that penetrate skin or mucosa, such as needles and surgical knives) must be heat-sterilized or disposable. Although they do not penetrate mucosa, handpieces are considered to be critical items. Semicritical items (ie, those that touch mucosa and/or non-intact skin, such as intraoral film holders) should also be heat-sterilized. If a semicritical item would be damaged by heat, then using a high-level disinfection is an option.

Instrument processing should take place in a central area dedicated to this activity. Provision should be made to prevent contaminated instruments from coming into contact with sterilized instruments. Instruments should be transported to the sterilization area in a puncture-proof container. There should be a specially designated "dirty" area in which the contaminated instruments are placed. This area should be physically separate from the "clean" area where sterilized instruments are located. If there will be a delay in processing the instruments, they should be placed in a holding solution to prevent blood and OPIM from drying on the surface.

Presterilization cleaning

All instruments must be thoroughly cleaned before sterilization. Ideally, this should be done with automated equipment. It is desirable to minimize the handling of instruments by DHCP. It is helpful to use instrument cassettes as these facilitate instrument processing and setup. Following decontamination of the instruments, the cassettes should be properly wrapped and dated. Indicator tape should be used to provide some assurance that proper operating temperature has been reached.

Steam sterilization process

The steam autoclave is the most popular means of sterilizing dental instruments. When using the autoclave, proper time and temperature settings must be used. Normally, autoclave use involves a temperature of 121°C at a pressure of 15 lbs for a period of 20 minutes [20]. Packaging material must permit the penetration of steam; overloading of the autoclave must be avoided. Mechanical, chemical, and biological monitors should be used (per manufacturer's instructions) to monitor the effectiveness of the sterilization process. Temperature and pressure gauges should also be observed during operation. The use of color-change autoclave tape may provide an early warning of an equipment malfunction. The most reliable method of monitoring sterilization efficacy involves biological indicators, often referred to as spore tests. Spore tests should be performed at least weekly. Every load containing implantable materials should be monitored biologically. In the event of a positive spore test, a standard protocol must be followed (Box 1).

Instrument storage

Following sterilization, instrument packs must be stored in a clean, dry area. This should be physically separated from the area in which contaminated instruments are processed. All packages should be marked with

Box 1. Protocol for positive spore test

- Affected instruments must be recalled and resterilized
- Remove autoclave from service
- Review process to identify possible operator error (eg, packaging, loading, monitoring)
- Retest unit with biological indicator and control
- If unit fails second test, affected instruments should be pulled from storage and resterilized with alternate autoclave
- If repeat test is negative and chemical/mechanical indicators satisfactory, place unit back in service
- Incident should be documented in sterilization log

a date of sterilization. Dating the packages will permit their retrieval in the event of a positive spore test. Instruments may be stored indefinitely, as long as the packaging remains intact.

Flash sterilization

"Flash sterilization" refers to the sterilization of unwrapped instruments for immediate use. This type of sterilization cycle should only be used after the instruments have been thoroughly cleaned. Autoclave gauges should be monitored for the correct temperature and pressure; a drying cycle should be included to facilitate aseptic transfer to the operatory.

Other methods of sterilization

Obviously, there are a number of other sterilization methods in use. These include chemical vapor and dry heat. Chemical vapor units cause less corrosion than the steam autoclave. Instruments must be dried before processing, however, and this is inconvenient. Dry heat is used on materials that cannot be subjected to moist heat. The dry heat process takes a longer time and requires higher temperatures than does autoclaving, however. Dry heat does not penetrate as well as steam, and will often cause charring of surgical towels. Other chemicals have also found useful in dental sterilization. Some liquid germicides are classified by the FDA as "sterilants" and they can be used on heat-sensitive critical and semicritical instruments. These agents (eg, glutaraldehyde) require prolonged immersion times (eg, 12 hours) and cannot be easily monitored. For these reasons, they are infrequently used in dental practices for the sterilization of instruments. Instead, these toxic compounds find limited use primarily as high-level disinfection of semicritical items.

Dental unit waterlines and surgical irrigation

Effluent from many dental offices does not meet the minimum EPA standards for drinking water quality (ie, ≤500 CFU/mL). As many as 200,000 CFU/mL have been recovered within days of installing new dental unit waterline (DUW) tubing [21]. This is due to biofilm formation in the tubing of dental units. The organisms populate the inner surface of the tubing in a matrix-enclosed community and are difficult to eradicate. Organisms from the biofilm are released during treatment and may be ingested or aspirated by the patient. The health implications of this phenomenon have not been elucidated, but there is the potential for disease transmission, particularly in susceptible hosts [22].

Dental units may be classified into "open" or "closed" systems based on their water source. Open units are connected to a municipal water supply, while closed systems (also known as "self-contained" systems) use a refillable reservoir attached to the unit. Dentists sometimes erroneously refer to closed units as "sterile water units", but the water from such units is not sterile even if sterile water is used to fill the reservoir.

The CDC states that DUW effluent must meet EPA drinking water standards. These standards specify that potable water contain less than 500 CFU of bacteria per milliliter. A requirement for periodic monitoring of the DUW effluent seems to be implied because microbial testing is the only way to determine if the effluent is acceptable. The effluent from closed systems can often be rendered acceptable by using a regimen of commercially available products [23,24]. The manufacturer can provide recommendations as to which products are compatible with specific units.

Open systems are more problematic, however. It is has been recommended that these units be flushed for varying periods, but this recommendation has not proven universally effective in the majority of related studies. There has been interest in the use of waterline tubing that possesses antimicrobial properties, but there is no consensus on the best way to solve this problem.

Surgical and endodontic irrigation require the use of sterile irrigating solution. It is not acceptable to use water from the air-water syringe or dental handpiece spray for this purpose.

Boil water advisories are issued when public water supplies exceed the threshold for microbial contamination. In such cases, water from the municipal water supply must not be used in dental units or patient care, nor should it be used for handwashing by DHCP. Alcohol-based handrub may be substituted for handwashing. When the advisory is lifted, obtain guidance from your local public health authority. If no guidance is provided, then flush all dental unit waterlines for 5 minutes before patient care [1] The manufacturer of the specific unit will provide further instructions on disinfecting waterlines.

Miscellaneous considerations

Dental handpieces

No handpiece should be used unless it is capable of withstanding heat sterilization. Potentially infectious material is often retracted into the interior of the handpiece, where it is difficult to remove. Therefore, high-speed handpieces (and other similar devices that enter the patient's mouth and are connected to the dental unit waterlines) should be run for approximately 20–30 seconds to clear the lines [1].

Dental evacuation systems

Patients should be instructed not to close their lips around saliva ejector tips because this may result in material from the suction system entering the mouth (ie, backflow). Saliva ejector and high-volume evacuation valves should be removable and sterilizable, particularly if the unit is used for surgical procedures. If this is not feasible, the valves should be cleaned thoroughly with an intermediate-level EPA-registered hospital disinfectant.

Parenteral medications

Parenteral medications pose special hazards because they are injected directly into the patient's body. To reduce the possibility of contamination, single-dose vials should be used whenever possible. If multi-use vials are used, the medications should be "drawn up" at a site distant from the actual treatment area. Before drawing up medications, the diaphragm (rubber top) should be thoroughly wiped with 70% alcohol and permitted to dry or wiped dry with a sterile gauze sponge. The vial should be kept stored in a secure, locked area where it is not subject to aerosols that might contaminate the top. Such vials should never be kept in treatment rooms or near ultrasonic cleaners in sterilization areas.

Quality assurance and program evaluation

Quality assurance (QA) is an important aspect of health care delivery. Employers are required to monitor the effectiveness of their programs and make changes accordingly. For example, if there is an increase in the number of percutaneous injuries, a cause should be sought. Is one employee responsible? Are employees recapping needles in an unsafe manner? Could the use of self-retracting needles reduce this risk? A record of all occupational exposures must be kept by the employer. Percutaneous exposures should be followed by immediate incident analysis to determine the proximate cause of the exposure and how recurrences can best be prevented.

Preventing recurrences is particularly important. The Needlestick Safety Act (P.L. 106-430) requires employers to periodically evaluate commercially available safety devices (eg, self-retracting needles) to determine whether they are suitable for use in the clinical environment. This evaluation process must include non-managerial employees who are involved in delivering patient care. This requirement could be best met via periodic meetings with the SIC officer or practice owner(s), but employees could also make suggestions. A trial use of a particular device may also be appropriate. Regardless of the nature of the process, it should be documented in the infection control plan.

The use of standardized, written IC protocols should also be considered a QA mechanism. Protocols should be posted in clinical areas where they can be referred to frequently. They should be laminated to prevent damage from liquids and permit easy surface disinfection.

Periodic staff meetings should be held to update training and discuss general IC and safety issues. Autoclaves should be routinely tested with an appropriate biological indicator and a log kept of the results. Autoclave failures can occur from a variety of causes, most notably leaking door gaskets. Processed instruments should be dated so that affected kits can be pulled from storage and resterilized. Each office should have clearly stated policy of autoclave monitoring, as well as a written protocol to be followed in the event of autoclave failure.

Summary

Infection control has had a major impact on dental practice over the last two decades. Further changes are inevitable as new threats emerge. New threats include the resurgence of various airborne diseases, such as tuberculosis, or the emergence of new diseases. It is incumbent upon dental health care workers to remain abreast of changes in the field so that they can continue to provide dental care while safeguarding the health of the public and themselves.

References

[1] Kohn W, Collins A, Cleveland J, et al. Guidelines for infection control in dental health-care settings—2003. Morbidity and Mortality Weekly Report 2003;52(No. RR-17).
[2] U.S. Department of Labor, Occupational Safety and Health Administration. 29 CFR Part 1910.1030. Occupational exposure to bloodborne pathogens, needlesticks and other sharps injuries: final rule. Federal Register 2001;66:5317–25.
[3] American Dental Association. Regulatory compliance manual. Chicago: American Dental Association; 1999.
[4] Bell DM. Occupational risk of human immunodeficiency virus infection in healthcare workers: an overview. Am J Med 1997;102:9–15.
[5] Dienstag JL, Isselbacher KJ. Acute viral hepatitis. In: Kasper DL, Braunwald E, Fauci AS, et al, editors. Harrison's principles of internal medicine, vol. 2. New York: McGraw-Hill; 2005. p. 1822–38.
[6] Alter MJ. Epidemiology and prevention of hepatitis B. Semin Liver Dis 2003;23:39–46.

[7] Dienstag JL, Isselbacher KJ. Chronic hepatitis. In: Kasper DL, Braunwald E, Fauci AS, et al, editors. Harrison's principles of internal medicine, vol. 2. New York: McGraw-Hill; 2005. p. 1844–55.
[8] Alter MJ. The epidemiology of acute and chronic hepatitis C. Clinics in Liver Disease 2003; 1(3):559–68, vi–vii.
[9] Alter MJ. Epidemiology of hepatitis C virus infection. World J Gastroenterol 2007;13: 2436–41.
[10] Shepard CW, Finelli L, Alter MJ. Global epidemiology of hepatitis C virus infection. Lancet Infect Dis 2005;5:558–67.
[11] Wasley A, Alter MJ. Epidemiology of hepatitis C: geographic differences and temporal trends. Semin Liver Dis 2000;20:1–16.
[12] Fauci AS. The AIDS epidemic—considerations for the 21st century. N Engl J Med 1999;341: 1046–50.
[13] Fauci AS, Lane HC. Human immunodeficiency virus disease: AIDS and related disorders. In: Kasper DL, Braunwald E, Fauci AS, et al, editors. Harrison's principles of internal medicine, vol. 1. New York: McGraw-Hill; 2005. p. 1076–139.
[14] Cegielski JP, Chin DP, Espinal MA, et al. The global tuberculosis situation. Progress and problems in the 20th century, prospects for the 21st century. Infect Dis Clin North Am 2002;16:1–58.
[15] Hopewell PC, Jasmer RM. Overview of clinical tuberculosis. In: Cole ST, Eisenach KD, McMurray DN, et al, editors. Tubculosis and the tubercle Bacillus. Washington: American Society for Microbiology Press; 2005.
[16] Raviglione MC, O'Brien RJ. Tuberculosis. In: Kasper DL, Braunwald E, Fauci AS, et al, editors. Harrison's principles of internal medicine, vol. 1. New York: McGraw-Hill; 2005. p. 953–66.
[17] Shah NS, Wright A, Bai GH, et al. Worldwide emergence of extensively drug-resistant tuberculosis. Emerg Infect Dis 2007;13:380–7.
[18] Wells CD, Cegielski JP, Nelson LJ, et al. HIV infection and multidrug-resistant tuberculosis: the perfect storm. J Infect Dis 2007;196(Suppl 1):S86–107.
[19] Prusiner SB. Prion biology and diseases. 2nd edition. Cold Spring Harbor (NY): Cold Spring Harbor Laboratory Press; 2004.
[20] Molinari JA, Rosen S, Runnells RR. Heat sterilization and monitoring. In: Cottone JA, Terezhalmy GT, Molinari JA, editors. Practical infection control in dentistry. 2nd edition. Media (PA): Williams and Wilkins; 1996.
[21] American Dental Association. Dental unit waterline quality. Available at: http://www.ada.org/prof/resources/topics/waterlines/art_cleaning_waterlines.pdf. Accessed April 8, 2008.
[22] Depaola LG, Mangan D, Mills SE, et al. A review of the science regarding dental unit waterlines. J Am Dent Assoc 2002;133:1199–206 [quiz: 1260].
[23] Linger JB, Molinari JA, Forbes WC, et al. Evaluation of a hydrogen peroxide disinfectant for dental unit waterlines. J Am Dent Assoc 2001;132:1287–91.
[24] McDowell JW, Paulson DS, Mitchell JA. A simulated-use evaluation of a strategy for preventing biofilm formation in dental unit waterlines. J Am Dent Assoc 2004;135:799–805.

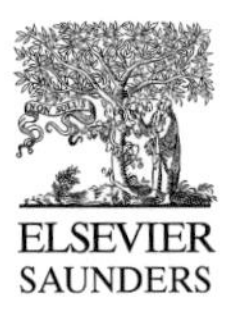

Dent Clin N Am 52 (2008) 629–639

THE DENTAL
CLINICS
OF NORTH AMERICA

Regulatory Compliance in the Dental Office

Mark V. Thomas, DMD[a,*], Glena Jarboe[b], Robert Q. Frazer, DDS[c]

[a]*Division of Periodontology, University of Kentucky, College of Dentistry, 800 Rose Street, Lexington, KY 40536-0297, USA*

[b]*University of Kentucky, College of Dentistry, 800 Rose Street, Room M 128, Lexington, KY 40536-0297, USA*

[c]*Division of Prosthodontics, University of Kentucky, College of Dentistry, 800 Rose Street, Lexington, KY 40536-0297, USA*

Regulatory compliance in the dental office

Dentists in the private sector, as well as their academic counterparts, must comply with a variety of federal, state, and local regulations. The scope of this regulation ranges from specifying who may engage in the practice of dentistry to the disposition of extracted teeth. In this review, we describe some of the requirements imposed by various regulatory agencies. Because of the importance of state and local oversight, each clinician must determine what state and local requirements exist for them. In some cases, the requirements may be virtually identical to the federal standard (as in the case of many states' Occupational Safety and Health Administration [OSHA] requirements). However, a number of states have enacted various regulations that are more stringent than the federal versions. It is necessary, therefore, to seek appropriate local counsel regarding applicable statutes and regulations. State dental societies are often a good place to begin this search. (The issue of infection control is described in a different article in this volume.)

The alphabet soup of regulatory compliance

Dentists often refer to infection control information as "OSHA" information. OSHA was, in fact, responsible for some of the earliest standards for the dental workplace. OSHA's mission is the protection of the employee

* Corresponding author.
E-mail address: mvthom0@uky.edu (M.V. Thomas).

doi:10.1016/j.cden.2008.02.003 *dental.theclinics.com*

and its standards reflect that emphasis. Although OSHA now plays a vital role in infection control in dentistry, it is not the only agency with an interest in infection control.

The Centers for Disease Control and Prevention (CDC), for example, have a broader mandate: the CDC is concerned with safeguarding the public's health. Obviously, this mandate is not confined to employees of dentists, but includes dentists, staff members, patients, and the public-at-large. Within the CDC is the National Institute for Occupational Safety and Health (NIOSH). Both NIOSH and OSHA were created by the Occupational Safety and Health Act of 1970. OSHA is charged with the development and enforcement of workplace safety and health regulations; NIOSH is responsible for improving workplace safety through research, education, and training in occupational safety and health.

Other agencies have some regulatory oversight of or interest in the dental health care industry, including the Environmental Protection Agency (EPA), which has an interest in hazardous waste and drinking water standards (which have been applied to dental unit waterline effluent lately). State and local public health authorities often have regulations that are more stringent than the federal standards. The more stringent standards take precedence over federal standards in that case. For that reason, the practitioner should always consult with local and state authorities to determine the applicable regulations for their jurisdiction.

All of the above-mentioned federal agencies have Web sites that are well-organized and informative. (Web sites include: www.osha.gov; www.cdc.gov; and www.epa.gov.) These Web sites have search features; most of the Web sites have publications or position papers on various topics that can be downloaded at no charge. These Web sites should be consulted as one of the first strategies when seeking information regarding regulatory compliance issues.

The American Dental Association (ADA) is also a good source of reliable information, as are many state and local dental societies. The ADA publishes a *Regulatory Compliance Manual* which is updated frequently [1]. The manual is a good, comprehensive reference and it is highly recommended.

Hazardous waste

Amalgam waste

The presence of mercury in amalgam has made it a source of concern for those charged with reducing mercury in the environment. Amalgam waste can be separated into contact and noncontact waste [2,3]. Contact waste is that amalgam waste that has been in contact with a patient's blood or body fluids. This would include amalgam that is in extracted teeth, plus that which is removed during restorative procedures. Noncontact waste has not been in a patient's mouth or exposed to blood or OPIM. Amalgam recyclers may treat these types of waste separately (and some may refuse to accept contact waste). It is prudent, therefore, to keep these wastes separated in the office.

The mercury found in amalgam is in a bound form. The environmental threat posed by such material is not entirely clear because the mercury is in a more inert form than some other sources of mercury. Nevertheless, there is legitimate concern that the improper disposal of amalgam may add to the overall mercury burden of the environment. Environmental mercury may eventually accumulate in fish that are then consumed by animals or humans.

Some of the environmental mercury burden is due to the release of mercury vapor. This will happen when amalgam is heated. For this reason, amalgam scrap and amalgam-containing extracted teeth should never be placed in sharps containers or in biohazard bags that are to be incinerated. Instead, all amalgam (including that found in extracted teeth) should be recycled. This includes amalgam scrap from evacuator traps and empty amalgam capsules. Although bulk mercury dispensers were formerly used by dentists, the ADA strongly recommends that bulk mercury dispensers be avoided in favor of precapsulated amalgam alloys.

A special concern may exist when plumbing work is needed in the dental office. Amalgam may be found in drainpipes and traps. Although this is considered to be largely inert and immobile, particles may dislodged by demolition or plumbing work. The ADA has published guidelines to aid in dealing with this potential problem [2,3].

A number of companies provide amalgam recycling services. It is important to pick a stable company with a good reputation. There are many laws governing the disposal of hazardous substances. It is incumbent upon the recycler to comply with these statutes and to indemnify the customer for the recycler's errors or omissions. The regulation of hazardous wastes involves "cradle-to-grave" responsibility that was established by the extensive and complex provisions of the Resource Conservation and Recovery Act (RCRA). The regulations are focused primarily on the prevention of pollution and the Comprehensive Environmental Response, Compensation, and Liability Act (CERCLA). They emphasize corrective, retrospective action such as cleanup of contaminated sites [4].

Silver waste

Silver waste is found in spent processing solutions in the form of silver thiosulfate complexes. Silver waste is regulated at the state and local level. Many municipalities and state governments have enacted regulations governing the disposal of this material because it often ends up in wastewater effluent. As in most other areas of regulatory compliance, the practitioner must determine the applicable local regulations and act accordingly. There are a number of options for recycling of spent solution, including the use of a commercial recycling service to pick up the used fixer.

Lead foil

Lead foil is used in many types of dental radiographic film. Lead is considered a hazardous material and should be recycled, rather than disposed of in regular waste [1]. With the increasing use of digital radiography, the significance of lead and silver waste in dentistry will diminish.

Volatile organic solvents and other materials

Biopsy containers must be kept tightly sealed, as they usually contain formalin or some other toxic tissue preservative. The containers must be clearly marked with the universal biohazard symbol, but they should also be labeled as to chemical content. If such containers are kept in the office, it will be necessary to have Material Safety Data Sheets (MSDSs) for the fixative used. Other potentially hazardous organic chemicals include methyl methacrylate monomer. This, and similar, materials will require special handling and disposal.

Regulated medical waste

Medical waste is a by-product of patient care. Waste generated in the dental office can be separated into regulated and nonregulated medical waste (Box 1). Many studies have demonstrated that general medical waste

Box 1. Regulated and nonregulated medical waste (from CDC guidelines)

Nonregulated waste

- General waste = residential waste
- Discard in regular trash
- Examples include: gloves; masks; gowns; lightly soiled gauze or cotton rolls; and environmental barriers

Regulated waste

- A limited subset of all medical waste
- Requires special storage, handling, and disposal
- Examples include: gauze saturated with blood; extracted teeth; sharps; and human tissue

Note: UKCD protocols are stricter, calling for all blood-contaminated material to be treated as regulated medical waste.

from hospitals (similar to that generated by a dental facility) is no more infective than normal household waste [5]. The CDC states that the "majority of soiled items in dental offices are general medical waste and thus can be disposed of with ordinary waste." Examples include used gloves, masks, gowns, lightly soiled gauze or cotton rolls, and environmental barriers (eg, plastic sheets and bags) used to cover equipment during treatment." While it is true that any item that has had contact with blood is potentially infective, the CDC further states that "treating all such waste as infective is neither necessary nor practical" [5].

Regulated medical waste, on the other hand, carries some theoretic but indeterminate risk and is, therefore, subject to special rules governing storage, transportation, and disposal. Examples of such waste include extracted teeth, sharps (blades, burs, needles), excised tissues, and materials that are saturated with blood or bodily fluids or OPIM. Sharps should be placed in a purpose-built, color-coded, puncture-resistant container that is prominently marked with the universal biohazard symbol. Nonsharp regulated waste may be safely placed in a heavy gauge, leak-proof bag (Fig. 1). Such bags should be securely closed before transport. Sharps containers should also have tight-fitting, secure lids that permit safe transportation to a disposal facility.

The disposal of such regulated medical waste generally falls under the purview of state agencies, although the EPA also has an interest in these activities. In 1991, Congress passed the Medical Waste Tracking Act (MWTA). This was done in response to the disquieting appearance of medical waste, including syringes, on several East Coast beaches. This problem received a great deal of attention from the media because the occurrence

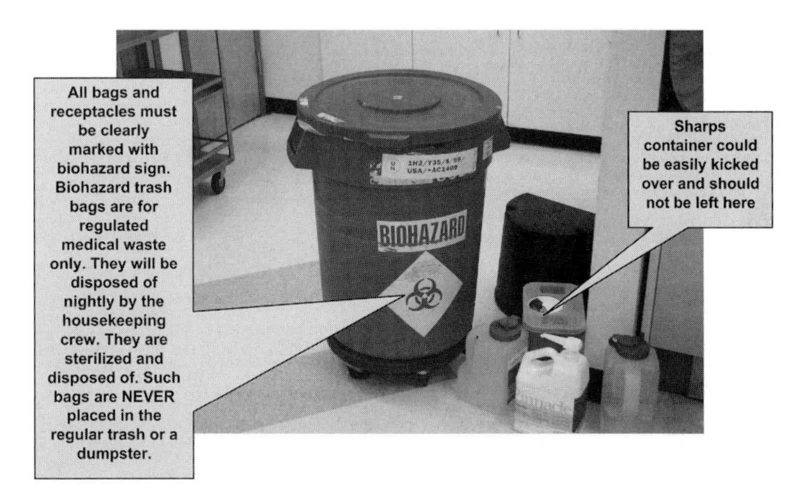

Fig. 1. Nonsharp medical waste must be disposed of in designated receptacles containing special red bags.

coincided with increasing public awareness of the AIDS epidemic. The MWTA required that medical wastes be defined and established a cradle-to-grave tracking system. Responsibility for the latter resides with the generator of the waste (ie, the dental office or other entity that generated the waste in the first place). The MWTA also established standards for packaging, labeling, and storing regulated medical waste. Most authority in this area resides with state and local authorities. Since regulations may vary in different jurisdictions, dentists should become familiar with all local and state regulations that pertain in their area.

Most waste generated by dental offices is not regulated medical waste. According to the EPA, "infectious waste" is waste that "contains pathogens with sufficient virulence and quantity so that exposure to the waste by a susceptible host could result in an infectious disease." Most of the waste generated in dental offices does not meet these criteria. An estimated 1% to 2% of the waste generated in dental offices is actually regulated medical waste. This would include blood-soaked gauze, extracted teeth, discarded sharps, and human tissue. The actual disease-causing potential of such waste is subject to debate. The EPA concluded that the disease-causing potential of medical waste is greatest at the point of generation and naturally tapers off after that point. Thus, risk to the general public of disease caused by exposure to medical waste is likely to be much lower than risk for the occupationally-exposed individual [6].

Most medical waste is incinerated. All generators of medical waste (including dental offices) should contract with a service provider who will pick up the waste and transport it in a safe manner to a site where it will be incinerated. New regulations that govern emissions from medical waste incineration (MWI) have been promulgated by the EPA. Due to the impact of these new rules, it is likely that many current incinerators will be shut down over the next several years. Providers will likely use alternative methods of compliance, including thermal methods, steam sterilization, electropyrolysis, and chemo-mechanical systems. The economic impact of these new processes is difficult to predict. States have their own agencies that oversee medical waste disposal. The EPA Web site has a Web page entitled "State Medical Waste Programs" with easy-to-use links to all state waste management agencies.

Proper handling of medical waste

Appropriate provisions must be made for the handling and disposal of regulated medical waste. Discarded sharps must be placed in a puncture-resistant container. Such containers must be clearly marked and should be near the point of use of the sharps. Nonsharp regulated medical waste (such as blood-soaked gauze) should be placed in a leak-resistant biohazard bag. The external surface of the bag must not be contaminated or it must be placed in a second bag.

Contaminated liquid waste

Liquid medical waste, including blood, can be poured into a drain connected to the public sanitary sewer system, in compliance with local and state regulations. When pouring large quantities of liquid, extreme care should be exercised and adequate personal protective equipment (PPE) should be worn, including a face shield.

Extracted teeth

Extracted teeth should be disposed of as medical waste unless returned to the patient or used for educational purposes. Teeth that are to be used for educational purposes should first be heat-sterilized (unless they contain amalgam). Amalgam-containing teeth must be cleaned and placed in a leak-proof , puncture-proof container marked with biohazard symbol. Extracted teeth containing amalgam must not be placed with medical waste that is to be incinerated, due to the likelihood that mercury vapor will be released. The ADA recommends that amalgam-containing teeth be recycled using the service provider that recycles your amalgam.

Ultimate disposal of medical waste

It is recommended that all offices contract with a reputable vendor for disposal of regulated medical waste. Such vendors should be reputable and stable, because cradle-to-grave liability may exist. The ADA recommends that that dentists ask such vendors if they will indemnify the practice owner against future legal liability. Criminal and civil penalties can be substantial in this area of regulatory compliance, so prudence should be used in evaluating a waste management program. Given the potential liability, dentists may wish to have an attorney review any contracts with waste management companies.

Record-keeping

Records of regulated waste disposal should be kept for a minimum of three years, but given the potential liability, it may be prudent to keep them for much longer. Most dental offices fall into the category of "small generators" which are defined as those producing less than 50 pounds per month (or perhaps less in some jurisdictions). Small generators may have less stringent record-keeping requirements, but this must be verified with local and state authorities. Regardless, it may be best to err on the side of caution with respect to such records. They generally do not require much space to store.

Hazard communication

All employers must identify hazardous chemicals present in the workplace. This information must be communicated to employees, using a combination of signage and more detailed product descriptions.

Signage/labeling requirements

All hazardous chemicals present in the workplace must be clearly labeled as to the nature of the hazard. For example, alcohol is present in many offices and does present several types of hazards, including flammability. Therefore, containers of alcohol should be labeled as to their contents (ie, "isopropyl alcohol") and the nature of the hazard(s) (eg, the term "flammable" or a universally understood symbol, such as flames). Information about individual chemicals hazards is available from a number of resources, including the NIOSH *Pocket Guide to Chemical Hazards*. This is available on the NIOSH Web site (http://www.cdc.gov/niosh/npg/) and it has an exhaustive alphabetical list of chemicals. It is not necessary that dental offices create their own labels. The labels should be present on the container as obtained from the manufacturer.

If the dental health care practitioner (DHCP) transfers the material to another container, however, this second container must be clearly labeled with the name and hazards associated with the chemical. This would be the case, for example, when surface disinfectant is dispensed from a large container into smaller spray bottles. These smaller containers must be labeled appropriately. The only exception to this rule is when the material transferred to the secondary container is to be used immediately. In any case, the label should contain the name of the product, the generic or chemical name, hazard warnings, and the manufacturer's name (along with appropriate contact information). If a product is regulated by the FDA or by the EPA, rather than by OSHA, then similar, but somewhat different, rules apply.

Hazard communication training

The individual office should have a specific hazard communication program. This should include a list of hazardous chemicals found in the office. This list should be updated when a new chemical is introduced. The office must maintain a current library of MSDSs. An MSDS must be available for each chemical found in the office and should be accessible to employees. Employees should receive training specific to the office. They should be familiar with the location and use of the MSDS library, the hazard communication signage in use, and knowledge of the hazard categories (such as hazards common to flammable or corrosive materials). New training is not required every time a new chemical is introduced into the workplace, but training is required when a new hazard is present. For example, consider the unlikely case of an office that has no flammable materials on hand, but then decides to introduce the organic solvent acetone. A quick check of the online NIOSH Pocket Guide to Chemical Hazards or (more likely) the MSDS indicates that this is a flammable material, thereby making it mandatory to train all employees in the hazards, handling, and storage of such agents.

As with all OSHA-mandated training, records should be kept of training sessions, topics covered, and those in attendance. These records should be part of the employee's individual training record.

General safety

With all of the emphasis on specific issues in regulatory compliance (eg, the Bloodborne Pathogens Standard), it is all too easy to forget more mundane safety considerations. These considerations might be termed general industrial safety issues, and include fire safety programs. All offices should have an evacuation plan in the event of fire or, in some areas, severe weather. Staff should know where exits are and where to meet after evacuation. There should be a protocol to be followed when a fire is discovered. Similarly, some policy should exist regarding the use of fire extinguishers. If extinguishers are available, staff should receive training in their use. Extinguishers should be checked periodically to ensure they are fully charged.

Many operations in the dental laboratory involve cutting and grinding operations. These require the use of personal protective equipment, even if the material is not contaminated with blood and body fluids. Safety glasses with eyeshields should be worn when performing such operations. Full face shields may be required for some procedures. Grinding on or working with gypsum products is potentially hazardous because of the calcium sulfate powder and silicates contained in such material. The hazards include various respiratory disorders, including silicosis. It is recommended that safety glasses and a suitable respirator be worn when working with such material. Many other materials used in the dental laboratory present potential hazards, including pickling solutions, various organic compounds (eg, methyl methacrylate), and gases used for soldering and casting. The relevant MSDS sheets should provide information on the safe handling of these materials.

Chemicals used in the processing of radiographic film are also hazardous. Protective eyewear should be used and skin contact should be avoided by using suitable gloves and other PPE. Such materials should be stored in clearly labeled containers with tightly sealed tops. Ionizing radiation obviously presents a potential risk to staff and patients. Practitioners should use best practices to reduce exposure, such as adequate collimation, lead shielding, standardized film exposure techniques and processing methods (to reduce the need for re-takes), and dosimetry badges. Many jurisdictions require initial and periodic inspections of devices that produce ionizing radiation. Practitioners should remain abreast of and adhere to the latest guidelines regarding the indications for diagnostic imaging [7].

Some studies have suggested that occupational exposure to nitrous oxide may present a health hazard to employees, especially women who are pregnant [8–10]. Scavenging systems are commercially available and are very effective in reducing the concentration of nitrous oxide in the ambient air [11,12]. Hoses, connections, bags, and other components should be checked regularly for leaks and tears that could lead to the escape of nitrous oxide into the office atmosphere. The scavenging system should be vented to the outside atmosphere; many local jurisdictions have regulations and building codes that address this issue. It may be prudent to consider the use of periodic monitoring of the general office atmosphere and the "personal" atmosphere in proximity to individual staff members who are actively treating sedated patients. Henderson and Matthews reported that episodic peak levels of nitrous oxide are much higher than the mean values over an entire work period [13].

Implantable device registry

Clinical science has greatly expanded our options for treatment of lost or missing tissues. This includes the implantation of various grafts and other forms of implants. Unfortunately, such devices have the potential to transmit disease or act as substrates upon which organisms can colonize. Additionally, patients may experience allergic reactions or other reactions to the materials contained in the implant. Although such materials undergo testing to ensure safety, problems may become obvious only after the material is used in clinical practice. Occasionally, the FDA will institute a recall of such material or devices. For example, in 2005 and 2006, the FDA issued recalls for allograft bone substitutes that had been improperly screened and/or harvested. A portion of the 2005 recall is reproduced below [14]:

> FDA and CDC recommend that implanting physicians inform their patients that they may have received tissue from a donor for whom an adequate donor eligibility determination was not performed. While the overall infectious risk is likely low, FDA and CDC recommend that physicians offer to provide patients access to appropriate infectious disease testing. The relevant communicable diseases for which a tissue donor is required to be tested are HIV-1 and 2 (the viruses that cause AIDS), hepatitis B virus, hepatitis C virus, and syphilis.

Note that the FDA directed dentists to contact patients who received these materials so that they could be tested. This implies that practitioners are able to identify all patients who received a certain type of implant or graft. It is obvious that not all charts could be reviewed to determine whether a given patient received a given material or not. Therefore, it is strongly suggested that all practitioners who use implantable materials of all types keep a log or registry of all patients receiving such materials, the date of implantation, its lot number, and the source of the material. While xenografts and allografts have a long track record of safety in dentistry and medicine, the potential exists for infectious disease transmission or other adverse effects. The patient's safety is entirely dependent upon the processors and distributors of these materials. Recent events suggest that clinicians should be vigilant about their sources for biological materials. Unanticipated adverse reactions to implantable materials or drugs should be reported to the manufacturer or distributor and, more importantly, to the

FDA. This can easily be done on the FDA's MedWatch Web site, http://www.fda.gov/medwatch/index.html.

Summary

The dental health care industry is regulated by a number of agencies. Despite a general trend toward de-regulation in certain industries, regulation of health care has increased. Many of the regulations have had a positive effect on improving safety in the workplace, while others have lessened the environmental impact of hazardous waste. Many of the federal, state, and local agencies charged with regulatory oversight have police powers and are capable of levying substantial fines. The dental practitioner must remain abreast of and responsive to changes in the regulatory environment. Fortunately, there are many sources of good information available from dental societies and regulatory agencies.

References

[1] American Dental Association. Regulatory compliance manual. Chicago (IL): American Dental Association; 1999.
[2] American Dental Association. Best management practices for amalgam waste. Chicago (IL): American Dental Association; 2005.
[3] American Dental Association. ADA guidelines on amalgam accumulations in dental office plumbing. Chicago (IL): American Dental Association; 2005. Available at: http://www.ada.org/prof/resources/positions/statements/amalgam_plumbing_guidelines.pdf. Accessed April 7, 2008.
[4] Sprankling JG, Weber GS. The law of hazardous wastes and toxic substances. St. Paul (MN): Thomson/West; 2007. p. 173–298.
[5] Centers for Disease Control and Prevention. Guidelines for infection control in dental health-care settings, 2003. MMWR 2003;52(No. RR-17):27.
[6] Environmental Protection Agency. Medical waste frequent questions. Available at: http://www.epa.gov/epaoswer/other/medical/mwfaqs.html. Accessed April 7, 2008.
[7] American Dental Association. ADA / FDA guide to patient selection for dental radiographs, 2005. Available at: http://www.fda.gov/cdrh/radhealth/adaxray.html. Accessed July, 2007.
[8] ADA Council on Scientific Affairs, ADA Council on Dental Practice. Nitrous oxide in the dental office. J Am Dent Assoc 1997;128(3):364–5.
[9] National Institute for Occupational Safety and Health. Control of nitrous oxide in dental operatories. Appl Occup Environ Hyg 1997;14(4):218–20.
[10] Howard WR. Nitrous oxide in the dental environment: assessing the risk, reducing the exposure. J Am Dent Assoc 1997;128(3):356–60.
[11] Hallonsten AL. Nitrous oxide scavenging in dental surgery. II. An evaluation of a local exhaust system. Swed Dent J 1982;6(5):215–23.
[12] Hallonsten AL. Nitrous oxide scavenging in dental surgery. I. A comparison of the efficiency of different scavenging devices. Swed Dent J 1982;6(5):203–13.
[13] Henderson KA, Matthews IP. Environmental monitoring of nitrous oxide during dental anaesthesia. Br Dent J 2000;188(11):617–9.
[14] U.S. Food and Drug Administration. FDA provides information on investigation into human tissue for transplantation, 2005. Available at: http://www.fda.gov/bbs/topics/NEWS/2005/NEW01249.html. Accessed March 28, 2008.

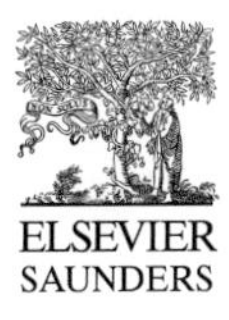

ELSEVIER
SAUNDERS

Dent Clin N Am 52 (2008) 641–651

THE DENTAL CLINICS OF NORTH AMERICA

Joint Commission of Accreditation of Healthcare Organization Accreditation for the Office-Based Oral and Maxillofacial Surgeon

Orville Palmer, MD, MPH, FRCSC[a,b,*], Phillip McIver, DDS[c]

[a]*Division of Otolaryngology, Head and Neck Surgery, Department of Surgery, Harlem Hospital Center, 506 Lenox Avenue, New York, NY 10037, USA*

[b]*Department of Otolaryngology, Columbia University College of Physicians and Surgeons, New York, NY, USA*

[c]*Department of Oral and Maxillofacial Surgery, Harlem Hospital Center, 506 Lenox Avenue, New York, NY 10037, USA*

Although general dentists do not get Joint Commission of Accreditation of Healthcare Organization (JCAHO) accreditation for their private offices, the authors believe that this article is relevant to the dental profession for many reasons. An increasing percentage of general dentists and dental specialists now practice in hospitals and other facilities that are accredited by the JCAHO and need an understanding of the accreditation process as they become leaders within these health care delivery systems. There is a national debate ongoing in the United States regarding the need for universal health care, which, if implemented, would bring along standards and regulations (understood by our medical colleagues) that the dental community also needs to understand. It is also a goal of the American Association of Oral and Maxillofacial Surgeons (AAOMS) to encourage members of their organization to seek JCAHO accreditation for their practices (some have done so), and the authors believe that periodontal practices could benefit from the information presented. Most of this article is geared to oral and maxillofacial surgeons (they have already started accrediting their offices) and, to some extent, periodontists because they are the surgical specialties

* Corresponding author. Division of Otolaryngology, Head and Neck Surgery, Department of Surgery, Harlem Hospital Center, 506 Lenox Avenue, New York, NY 10037.

E-mail address: odp3@columbia.edu (O. Palmer).

doi:10.1016/j.cden.2008.02.009 *dental.theclinics.com*

of dentistry. It is also intended for the general dental community, however. Even if one does not seek accreditation for his or her office, many of the goals and standards of the JCAHO are good for safe and effective health care delivery.

The delivery of safe high-quality care and services should be the goal of all patient care facilities. As oral and maxillofacial surgeons and periodontists increase, and continue to increase, the volume and complexity of surgical procedures performed in the office, it is imperative that we maintain the quality of care that the profession has upheld in the public eye for so many years [1]. Accreditation by a managed care agency is one definitive method through which an office-based surgery facility can attain the recognition of achieving an established standard and provide an internal "check and balance" system ensuring that a superior standard of care is being maintained. During 2000 in Florida, there were several unfavorable outcomes in the surgical office setting that sparked media attention to health and safety issues provided by office-based surgeons [2]. Although regulations were already in place in the hospital setting, the state legislation felt the demand to become involved in regulating office-based surgical care. Surgical specialties are at risk for receiving negative attention if the complexity and volume of office-based procedures outstrip the capacity of the office to provide appropriate resources and "back-up"—particularly during emergency situations. The possibility of less than desirable surgical outcomes can easily increase in this environment. It is therefore prudent to take active and reasonable measures to implement standards ensuring that quality care is being provided. Many of these standards have been established by various regulatory agencies and organizations, with the JCAHO being one of them.

A steady increase in the cost of in-hospital health care has resulted in an increased demand for often more affordable office-based surgery. It is estimated that 15% to 20% of all outpatient operations in the medical community are now being performed as office-based surgical procedures, and in oral and maxillofacial surgery, more than 90% of the procedures are performed in the office. As many surgical procedures steadily moved from hospitals to outpatient-based settings in the early 1980s, the transfer of the oversight functions, unfortunately, did not follow [3]. Many surgeons who could not get privileges in hospitals were able to practice in their offices. This was fairly common for cosmetic surgical procedures. State governments began to consider the need for standards to protect health consumers from inadequately trained practitioners, ill-equipped facilities, and preventable anesthesia-oriented incidents [3,4].

Oral surgeons have been among the leaders in the field of office-based surgery under general anesthesia. Third molar surgery has given the specialty its current stronghold on office-based surgery. The validity for the procedure has been well established, and this has allowed oral surgeons to become the model for other providers of office-based surgery. The removal of third molars in young adults has been a widely accepted preventive procedure proved to promote periodontal health in the second molar [5]. In addition, the supported indications for early third molar removal include systemic health considerations, prevention of odontogenic cysts, crowding of mandibular incisors, orthodontic considerations, and pericoronitis, to name a few [6]. A widely accepted trend has been to perform third molar surgery under office-based ambulatory anesthesia, allowing for patient comfort from anxiety through an often difficult surgical procedure. The worldwide acceptance of this practice has maintained a consistent high volume of office-based ambulatory surgery in the oral and maxillofacial surgery office setting. It is also important to consider patient satisfaction as an indication for quality care. Clinical trials in outcome assessment reveal that more than 90% of patients who have undergone oral surgery under local anesthesia, conscious sedation, or general anesthesia felt safe and reported a high level of satisfaction after surgery [7,8]. This has also established oral surgery practice as a model for conscious sedation in other medical specialties, such as colonoscopy and plastic surgery.

National patient safety goals

The national patient safety goals were initially created by the Joint Commission to improve patient safety in the hospital setting. These goals have been further developed into a useful tool for providing a safe environment for patients in the ambulatory care and office-based surgical setting. These goals can be applied specifically to the oral and maxillofacial surgery practice [9,10] and can also be modified for the larger general practice or multispecialty office.

The Joint Commission has implemented these goals, focusing on problematic areas in health care delivery, in the accreditation process and requirements. When an organization does not demonstrate implementation of a safety goal requirement, it is assigned a requirement for improvement similar to the requirement for improvement assigned to compliance with a standard. In the accreditation process, all requirements for improvement with regard to national patient safety goals must be addressed [10].

The national patient safety goals applicable to the oral and maxillofacial surgery office address problematic areas, such as the following:

1. Improving the accuracy of patient identification
2. Improving the effectiveness of communication among caregivers (accuracy of referral requests)
3. Improving the safety of using medications
4. Reducing the risk for health care–associated infections
5. Accurate and complete reconciliation of medications across the continuum of care
6. Reducing the risk for surgical fires

7. Encouraging patients' active involvement in their own care as a patient safety strategy
8. Universal protocol with regard to correct patient and surgery site identification at the time of surgery

A brief summary of each goal requirement is given here; the detailed goal description, rationale, implementation, and expectation of requirement can be found on the Joint Commission Web site [10].

Improving the accuracy of patient identification

Use at least two patient identifiers when providing care, treatment, or services to prevent patient errors in diagnosis and treatment. This is important in the practice with multiple doctors or in hospital practices in which charts may be switched.

Improving the effectiveness of communication among caregivers

It is important for general practitioners who refer patients to dental specialists that the request for service requested is clear. Wrong tooth extractions and other such errors can lead to embarrassment, malpractice suits, and irreversible harm to the patient. Likewise, surgeons and endodontists, for example, should be careful with referrals and communicate with the referrer if there is ever the slightest doubt.

Within the hospital setting or when communicating with nurses, clerks, or laboratory personnel, verify verbal or telephone orders by having the complete order or test result "read-back" by the receiving personnel. This promotes effective communication, and thus reduces critical errors in patient care. In addition, the standardization of abbreviations and assessment of timely reporting of critical test results are important. The Joint Commission recommends a "hand-off" approach to communication in which caregivers take time and opportunity to ask and respond to questions when changing shifts or transferring a patient to postanesthesia recovery areas.

Improving the safety of using medications

Review and identify sound-alike drugs, and provide an effective method of labeling all medications. Syringes used during intravenous sedation should be labeled.

Reducing the risk for health care–associated infections

An organization should be in absolute compliance with the World Health Organization (WHO) or Centers for Disease Control and Prevention (CDC) hand hygiene guidelines, thus decreasing the transmission of infectious agents from staff to patients. Nearly all states and jurisdictions in the United States require dentists to have proof of having completed a course in infection control as a part of being credentialed for licensure or renewal. Occupational Safety and Health Administration (OHSA) requirements for dental practice must also be in place, and supporting documents must be kept in the office.

Accurate and complete reconciliation of medications across the continuum of care

Communication of a complete list of current patient medications to compare with those ordered should be ensured in providing a continuum of patient care. An accurate and updated medication list should be maintained as a part of the medical history. Practitioners should be aware of drug interactions, and there are several handheld electronic devices that should be used to check for possible drug interactions when a new drug is being added.

Reducing the risk for surgical fires

Educate staff in maintaining and monitoring heat and fuel sources in consideration of timely patient intervention in the event of a surgical fire.

Encouraging patients' active involvement in their own treatment

Provide a method and means of communicating with the patient and patient's family regarding all aspects of treatment and services to be rendered. Involving patients in their own health care decisions improves acceptance of the proposed surgical procedure, alleviates misunderstandings, and prevents malpractice claims.

Universal protocol

Implement a preoperative verification process to prevent wrong site, wrong patient, and wrong procedure surgery. Review relevant documents, such as the patient consent, history and physical examination findings, relevant images before the start of the procedure, and implementation of a "time-out" protocol in which the procedure team provides final verification of patient and procedure. It is not required by the JCAHO that teeth be marked on the patient or on radiographs as part of the site verification process. Nevertheless, it is required that teeth to be extracted or treated be listed by numbers (1–32) in the patient's medical records. Implant sites can be marked on the radiographs.

Benefits of accreditation

Accreditation by the JCAHO should be viewed as a valuable accomplishment for a practice to attain. It is an intensive customized process with specific goals, value, and mission. Practices that are accredited have a marketing advantage as today's consumers shop for affordable superior health care. Many patients view accreditation as a seal of approval and a measure of professional achievement. In addition, accredited facilities are recognized nationally by third-party payers, health maintenance organizations, preferred provider organizations, government agencies, and employers who seek to select high-quality health care providers. Professional liability insurance carriers see it as an indicator of quality and do take special consideration in evaluating an organization applying for coverage, thus improving access to liability coverage. In addition, the cost of liability insurance decreases if an institution is accredited. Accreditation enhances staff recruitment and development. Finally, it provides management and organizational structure to maintain a high level of compliance with proved standards. In doing so, the Joint Commission acts as a guide to improving quality efforts [11,12]. At the state level, laws may be in place requiring providers to have accreditation that may be fulfilled by the Joint Commission process.

Joint Commission history

The Joint Commission is a private not-for-profit organization committed to continuously improving the safety and quality of medical care provided to the public by providing standards, survey evaluations, sentinel event alerts, professional consulting services, and related services that support performance improvement to health care organizations. In its main capacity as an accrediting body, the JCAHO currently evaluates and accredits 18,000 health care organizations, including hospitals, ambulatory surgery centers, outpatient facilities, health care networks, and clinical laboratories.

The first hospital inspections in the United States were performed by the American College of Surgeons (ACS) in 1918, based on the ACS Minimum Standard for Hospitals. In 1951, the ACS joined the American College of Physicians, the American Hospital Association, and the American Medical Association to form the Joint Commission on Accreditation of Hospitals (JCAH), an independent not-for-profit organization whose primary purpose was to provide voluntary accreditation. In 1952, the JCAH took over the hospital standardization program from the ACS, and in 1953, it published the JCAH Standards for Hospital Accreditation. With the passage of the Medicare Act in 1965, the role of the JCAH shifted, becoming more closely tied to the government. The law provided that hospitals accredited by the JCAH were deemed in compliance with most of the Medicare conditions of participation for hospitals, and thus were considered eligible to participate in the Medicare program [13]. In 1975, the JCAH broadened its reach by accrediting office-based surgical facilities and ambulatory health care facilities through the Accreditation Council for Ambulatory Healthcare, and in 2001, the Joint Commission introduced standards and a survey process for smaller office-based surgery practices. Today, more than 300 office-based surgery practices are accredited by the Joint Commission [13,14].

Accreditation is a voluntary process that does not take the place of licensure or certification but may act as a supplement or grounds on which to certify [14,15]. The accreditation process consists of an initial survey or early survey policy option, a self-evaluation study, and on-site observances and interviews by surveyors every 3 years. The group of surveyors consists of experienced health care professionals trained to provide expert advice and education.

To be eligible for accreditation by the Joint Commission, the practice must be located in the United States or its territories, or if outside the United States, it should be operated by the US government or under a charter of the US Congress.

A practice interested in accreditation for the first time by the Joint Commission or one that has not been unaccredited in the past 6 months is eligible for the initial survey.

The practice must be owned and operated by a physician (including dentists and podiatrists). Local anesthesia, general anesthesia, or sedation must be administered.

The practice must be composed of four or fewer licensed independent practitioners, whether at a single site or at multisites. The practice must identify the services addressed by the Joint Commission's standards that it provides and indicate which services are provided directly, under contract, versus those provided through some other arrangement [11,14]. The practice assesses and improves the quality of its services based on the review of the surveyors.

The cost of a typical 1-day survey is $5520 and an additional $2580 per extra day if a practice includes more than one site. The JCAHO requires that a facility post a public announcement requesting comments from the public before the survey. This step enables anyone who has information about an organization's compliance with the standards to request an interview with the surveyors at the time of the visit. After the survey, information regarding safety and quality of the practice is available to the public on a Web site [16].

The customized standards used by the Joint Commission for accreditation were developed by consultation with health care experts, providers, and researchers and with purchasers and consumers.

Tracer methodology

During the on-site visit, surveyors focus on evaluating actual care processes by tracer methodology, which traces patients through the care, treatment, and services they received, analyzing key operational systems in place that have a direct impact on the quality and safety of patient care. Unique to each practice are its clinical service groups (CSGs), which may include endoscopy, plastic surgery, ophthalmology, otolaryngology, or oral maxillofacial surgery. The tracer methodology is the premise on which the on-site survey is based. This may take the form of (1) individual tracer activity or (2) the individual-based system tracer activity.

The individual tracer activity is an evaluation methodology that traces a patient experience at the practice. The patients are chosen from the top CSGs for that practice or from patients related to topic, such as medication management or infection control. Based on the CSGs, an individual tracer would be identified. The tracer is then followed through the practice process. The surveyor looks at the management provided by each unit, program, or department and services and how these components interact with each other. Once the tracer is identified, the surveyor may then move to any point of encounter experienced by the tracer and get required information through interviews.

The individual-based system tracer activity looks more at systems and processes in the practice affecting a group of patients. The Joint Commission evaluates the various systems, processes, and structure of an office based on 14 different areas called priority focus areas. The priority focus areas are the following:

Assessment and care and services
Communication
Credentialed practitioners
Equipment use
Infection control
Information management
Medication management
Organizational structure
Orientation and training
Patient safety
Physical environment
Quality improvement expertise and activities
Rights and ethics
Staffing

The priority focus areas guide the surveyors in the compliance assessment, especially when individual-based tracer activities are undertaken [14]. In this type of evaluation, the surveyor evaluates the system. This differs from the individual tracer activity, in which an individual is followed through his or her stages of care.

In addition, the Joint Commission makes evaluations based on verbal and written information provided to the Joint Commission, on-site observations and interviews, and documents provided by the practice.

Unannounced surveys are also conducted. This normally takes place 9 to 30 months after the last day of the full survey. This is done by one surveyor over 1 day, and the practice is not charged for this survey. On request by a patient or staff member, or if a serious situation is identified in a practice that puts at risk the safety of the public, the Joint Commission may provide accreditation-related information to state, federal, or local governmental or licensing agencies.

Sentinel event

A sentinel event is an unsuspected occurrence involving a serious physical (loss of limb or vital function) or psychologic injury. As a part of its mission to provide safe and improving quality health care, the Joint Commission reviews the institution's response as it relates to sentinel events during the full survey or the random survey. Not all sentinel events occur because of a medical error.

There are four specific goals of a sentinel event policy:

1. To improve patient care and safety by recognizing and preventing these events
2. If a sentinel event occurs, the organization should learn from it and modify the institution policy and systems to prevent further occurrence.
3. To create strategies for future prevention
4. To keep the confidence of the public and the accredited institution in the accreditation process.

During the survey the organization is scored based on standardized performance-based protocols. The practice's process for responding to sentinel events is reviewed, and interviews of the practice's staff are conducted on their responsibilities for identifying, responding to, and reporting sentinel events.

During the accreditation process, the surveyors are discouraged from probing for a sentinel event not already known or reported to them. If such an event is identified at a survey, it is reported to practice leaders and reported formally to the Joint Commission. In the event of a sentinel event, a detailed root cause analysis and action plan should be prepared and be submitted within 45 day of the occurrence or becoming aware of the occurrence of the event. Failure to do so might affect the accreditation status outcome of the organization [14].

Decisions

After the on-site survey, the practice receives a report that outlines findings and any follow-up requirements for improvement that must be addressed to receive accreditation status. There are six possible decisions with clear conditions that lead to the respective outcomes:

1. Accreditation: the facility is in compliance with all acceptable set standards at the time of the survey or has addressed all requirements in an evidence of standards compliance report presented with 45 days after the JHACO issues the accreditation survey finding report.
2. Provisional accreditation: this is issued when after a 45-day posting of the accreditation survey finding report, the facility fails to address all the requirements for improvement.

3. Conditional accreditation: the facility is not in substantial compliance with the acceptable standards. This occurs when the facility is more than 1.5 to 3.0 SDs greater than the mean for noncompliant standards.
4. Preliminary denial of accreditation: this decision is subject to appeal. It occurs when the count of noncompliant standards exceeds 3.0 SDs. A practice that receives a decision of preliminary denial of accreditation has 10 business days to submit clarifying information demonstrating its compliance with one or more standards in question.
5. Denial of accreditation: all appeal opportunities have been exhausted.
6. Preliminary accreditation: the facility demonstrates compliance with preselected standards in the first of two surveys in the early survey policy option 1 [14].

The Joint Commission quality report provides information on an office-based surgery organization's accreditation information and on other organizations with which comparisons are made. It contains the following:

1. Accreditation decision date and accreditation of any other health care program within the organization
2. Any special awards or quality distinctions achieved specifically for office-based practice
3. Result of national safety goals displayed in survey against standard goals in effect
4. Overview of the accreditation process
5. Joint Commission history and the processes it uses to set standards and compliance
6. Care delivery issues addressed by the accreditation process, such as infection control and safety issues pertaining to medication administration

The Joint Commission quality report is made available to the public after the survey.

Summary

Office-based surgery has become a vital component of the practice of oral and maxillofacial surgeons and periodontists. It has enabled these specialties to provide needed service to patients in an outpatient setting, including the option of intravenous sedation. It is the stance of this article to promote professional oversight and quality assurance through accreditation by the Joint Commission to maintain a standard in the delivery of office-based surgical services, thus upholding the integrity of the profession in the clinical setting.

References

[1] ACS Board of Governors' Committee on Ambulatory Surgical Care. Guidelines for office-based surgery: quality assurance. Bull Am Coll Surg 1994;79(10):32–4.

[2] Florida Board of Medicine. Florida Department of Health moratorium alert (Tallahassee, FL: Florida Board of Medicine, Aug 10, 2000).
[3] JCAHO Board of Commissioners. Report of the special committee on outpatient (office-based) surgery. JCAHO.
[4] Franho F. State legislative coordinator, state laws and regulations for office based surgery. AORN J 2001;7(4):839–46.
[5] White R. Progress report on third molar clinical trials. J Oral Maxillofac Surg 2007;65: 377–83.
[6] Marciani R. Third molar removal: an overview of indications, imaging, evaluation, and assessment of risk. Oral Maxillofac Surg Clin North Am 2007;19(1):1–13.
[7] Perrott D, Yuen J, Andresen R, et al. Office-based ambulatory anesthesia: outcomes of clinical practice of oral and maxillofacial surgeons. J Oral Maxillofac Surg 2003;61:983–95.
[8] Coyle T, Helfrick J, Gonzalez M, et al. Office-based ambulatory anesthesia: factors that influence patient satisfaction or dissatisfaction with deep sedation/general anesthesia. J Oral Maxillofac Surg 2005;63:163–72.
[9] Assel L. The need for national patient safety goals for ambulatory surgery. J Oral Maxillofac Surg 2007;65:1–2.
[10] JCAHO Board of Commissioners. JCAHO 2008 ambulatory care and office-based surgery national patient safety goals. Available at: http://www.jointcommission.org/PatientSafety/NationalPatientSafetyGoals/08_amb_obs_npsgs.htm. Accessed August 15, 2007
[11] JCAHO Board of Commissioners. Benefits of Joint Commission accreditation. Available at: http://www.jointcommission.org/AboutUs/joint_commission_facts.htm. Accessed May 19, 2007.
[12] Haymen MR. Accreditation of the office-based surgical facility. Bull Am Coll Surg 1995; 80(8):8–11.
[13] Franko F. The important role of the Joint Commission. AORN J 2002;75(6):1179–82.
[14] JCAHO Board of Commissioners. Accreditation manual for office-based surgery practices. Oakbrook Terrace: Joint Commission on Accreditation of Health Care Organizations.
[15] Cericola SA. What is the credentialing process? Plast Surg Nurs 1996;16(4):257–8.
[16] JCAHO Board of Commissioners. Available at: www.qualitycheck.org. Accessed May 19, 2007.

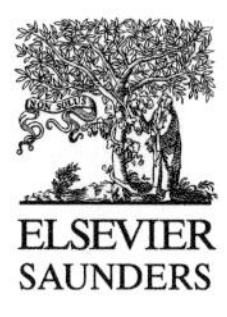

ELSEVIER
SAUNDERS

Dent Clin N Am 52 (2008) 653–668

THE DENTAL
CLINICS
OF NORTH AMERICA

Complying with the Occupational Safety and Health Administration: Guidelines for the Dental Office

Ricardo Boyce, DDS*, Justin Mull, DMD

Department of Dentistry/Oral Maxillofacial Surgery, The Brooklyn Hospital Center, 121 Dekalb Avenue, Brooklyn, NY 11201, USA

In 1970 more than 14,000 accidental deaths occurred in the workplace in the United States [1]. In an effort to reduce the number of injuries and deaths among United States workers, Congress passed legislation, termed the Occupational Safety and Health Act, that year establishing new workplace safety laws. The Occupational Safety and Health Administration (OSHA), created as a division of the Department of Labor, enacts workplace safety standards and oversees these standards. OSHA rules apply to dental clinics and all other privately owned places of work in the United States. Compliance with OSHA guidelines is mandatory for all owners of dental practices that employ dental personnel. Federal law requires OSHA annual training sessions on current OSHA regulations for all dental offices. Fines and penalties are imposed on employers who fail to meet OSHA standards. Dental practice owners are given an opportunity to redress shortfalls in workplace safety protocols and have the right to challenge any citations deemed unfair. The OSHA regulations are readily available and clearly stated in print and on-line formats. The American Dental Association (ADA) also publishes updated OSHA compliance standards for dental offices, available since 2003 through a link on the ADA Web site (http://www.osha.gov/dcsp/compliance_assistance/quickstarts/health_care.html) [2]. In dental clinics and in all places where dentists practice, OSHA protections are especially important to provide safeguards against biologic pathogen transmission and physical injuries, including needlesticks.

OSHA broadened its protections for workers in 1980 to reduce chemical and biologic risks to workers [3]. Employees, protected under OSHA regulations from exposure to such risks, cannot lose employment for calling

* Corresponding author.
E-mail address: raboycedds@yahoo.com (R. Boyce).

doi:10.1016/j.cden.2008.03.002

attention to workplace hazards. As a result of OSHA rules, the number of workplace deaths fell to fewer than 6000 by 2006, less than half of what it was in 1970 [4]. OSHA has helped reduce workplace fatalities by more than 60% and occupational injury and illness rates by 40% [5]. In two of the historically most dangerous industries, agriculture and construction, workplace injuries and deaths have been reduced dramatically [6]. In contrast, as a result of the increase in the number of health care workers, the number of workplace injuries for dentists are increasing [7]. The health care profession (with more than 12 millions workers) is the second fastest growing sector of the United States economy, and absolute numbers of injuries to health care workers continue to rise [8]. Injuries common to health care personnel include occupational hazards (such as needlestick injuries), exposure to blood-borne pathogens, back injuries, and workplace violence. Disability insurers report that one in three general dentists go on disability at some point during their careers. The regulations of OSHA are great in scope and also specific in areas, such as proper sterilization technique and protection from needlestick injuries. OSHA offices are located in every state in the United States and officials from OSHA monitor workplace safety through unannounced inspections. Certain states have OSHA programs with requirements that are more strict than federal OSHA requirements. Federal, state, and local OSHA officials issue citations and penalties to dental practices not in compliance with current OSHA regulations.

The Occupational Safety and Health Administration mandate

The OSHA mission for nearly 4 decades has been to ensure the safety and health of workers in the United States. OSHA standards are set and enforced through random, unannounced inspections of dental practices throughout the United States. OSHA workers, however, also provide training and education and partner with other associations, such as the ADA and the National Institute for Occupational Safety and Health (NIOSH) in an effort to improve workplace safety and the health of dental care practitioners and their staff. All workers in the dental field are covered by federal OSHA regulations or through one of the 26 OSHA-approved state-run programs. Some states, such as Connecticut, New Jersey, and New York, and the Virgin Islands have OSHA programs that cover state and local government dental practices only; federal OSHA rules apply to all private practices [9]. OSHA standards apply to dental practices in which the owner of a practice has one or more employees.

Occupational Safety and Health Administration standards

The general aim of OSHA standards is to maintain conditions and practices that protect dentists and auxiliary dental personnel from hazards in the patient care environment. The OSHA standards were established to promote workplace safety and are enforced through inspections, citations, and financial penalties. Through a combination of standards for safety equipment and workplace practices, OSHA aims to reduce risks to workers, including the risk for transmission of blood-borne illnesses. Practice owners and their employees must be familiar with and comply with OSHA standards and have personal protective equipment available for use in dental practices to promote safety and health for employees and patients.

Inspectors from OSHA may come to any health care facility or hospital in the United States and issue citations for improper infection control, construction safety, or other issues; in the past few years, OSHA citations have risen 32% [10]. The financial penalties for infractions that have put workers at risk have risen 75% [11]. The onus is on employers to understand the responsibilities outlined by OSHA and to comply with the government agency's standards. A poster advising dentists and dental auxiliary staff of job safety and health protection must be posted in dental offices. Posters 3165 in English and 3167 in Spanish are available on-line at http://www.osha.gov/Publications/osha3165.pdf or http://www.osha.gov/Publications/osha3167.pdf. Current OSHA standards are laid out clearly in publications available from OSHA on-line at www.osha.gov and through the mail, and OSHA established a toll-free call center telephone number in the early 1990s at (800) 321-OSHA (6742) for further assistance and incident reporting. The complete text of OSHA regulations applying to medical and dental offices may be found listed as Code 29 of the Code of Federal Regulations.

OSHA has a dental practice section on its Web site at www.osha.gov/SLTC/dentistry/standards.html. Although there are no specific OSHA standards for dentistry, there are many areas where general OSHA standards are particularly important (Table 1). Exposure to biologic, chemical, environmental, physical, and psychologic hazards are addressed in OSHA regulations. The OSHA Standard Industrial Classification system for general dentistry is Code 8021 and for dental laboratories, Code 8072 [5]. Where no specific standard for a given workplace condition in dental practice exists, the OSHA General Duty Clause applies. The Clause states, all employers "shall furnish... a place of employment which is free from

Table 1
General industry standards following specific standards often cited for dentistry

29 CFR 1910.1030	Blood-borne pathogens
29 CFR 1910.1200	Hazard communication
29 CFR 1910.1450	Occupational exposure to hazards
29 CFR 1910.151	Medical services and first aid
29 CFR 1910.134	Respiratory protection
29 CFR 1910.132	Personal protective equipment
29 CFR 1910.148	Formaldehyde
29 CFR 1910.157	Portable fire extinguishers
29 CFR 1910.105	Nitrous oxide

recognized hazards that are causing or are likely to cause death or serious physical harm to their employees" [12]. State OSHA regulations are as demanding as the federal standards. All dental offices must comply with standards specific to the dental profession included in Code 8021.

Universal precautions

OSHA regulations stress the implementation of universal precautions in clinics, operatories, and surgical suite settings. The workplace for oral surgeons, general dentists, and staff may contain many physical dangers. The possibility of exposure to pathogens through contact with patients exists with each patient contact. OSHA has established safety standards regarding blood-borne pathogens to protect against infection. The standards require an exposure plan, annually updated, which includes quick and accurate methods for the determination for an exposure. Lists of all employment activities in which there is increased risk for exposure to infectious materials also must be in place [13]. Paramount among the universal precautions is proper handwashing by health care workers. Employers are required by OSHA to provide employees with handwashing facilities or "where not possible, an antiseptic rinse or cleanser must be provided as a temporary means of hand sanitation" [14]. Effective antibacterial hand cleansers are available that may substitute for handwashing with soap and water. According to the OSHA standards, these hand sanitizers must be readily available, meaning that employees should not have to leave an examination room or operatory to obtain them.

When contact with potentially infectious materials, such as blood, occurs on keratinized skin, OSHA standards require immediate and thorough washing of the affected skin surface. When exposure has occurred to mucous membranes or eyes of the health care worker, OSHA mandates flushing the surfaces with water [15]. Universal precautions help minimize the risks of known methods of disease transmission. The eyes, mucous membranes of the nose and mouth, and areas of the hands that are not intact skin, as are present after a cut, are vulnerable areas for oral surgeons and other health care workers. Thus, eye protection, masks, and gloves have become standard attire while providing care where pathogen-containing fluids may be present. Eye and face protection meet requirements specified by the American National Standards Institute (ANSI) system.

Table 2 summarizes OSHA regulations for general practice offices and the timeline for implementation OSHA requirements.

Personal protective equipment

OSHA has the authority to enforce the ANSI standards, and all safety glasses goggles and face shields worn by employees under OSHA

Table 2
Occupational Safety and Health Administration regulations and timeline

Occupational Safety and Health Administration regulation	Timeline	Requirement/evaluation activity
Employee OSHA training	Annual	Employers are required to annually review all OSHA guidelines with employees and educate regarding updated infection control standards
Immunization programs	Year round	Availability of hepatitis B vaccination; employees who refuse must be given a declination statement. Annual review of personnel records to ensure up-to-date immunizations
Blood-borne pathogen exposure management	Year round	Postings regarding minimization of risks and postexposure guidelines must be made available to all employees and policies regarding exposure reporting must be explained to all employees
		Documentation of exposures and steps for exposure prevention
Workplace controls for percutaneous needle injuries	Year round	Disposable syringes and needles with safeguard closures and easily accessible sharps containers
Antiseptic rinses and cleansers	Year round	Availability of hand rinse and cleansers. Observe and document appropriate handwashing.
Evaluation and implementation of safer medical devices	Annual	Annual review of exposure control plan and implementation of newer and safer medical devices
Personal protective equipment	Year round	Protective eyewear, masks, and face shields must be available to the clinician during any procedure in which aerosol or airborne pathogens may be present
Proper handling and disposal of medical waste	Year round	Observe the safe disposal of regulated and nonregulated medical waste and appropriate preventive measures in place should hazardous situations occur
Health care–associated infections	Year round	Assess the circumstances resulting in a suspected transmission from patient to practitioner or vice versa and implement steps to reduce exposure risks

jurisdiction must meet the Z87.1 standard. The ANSI Z87.1 standards enforced by OSHA include mandatory requirements for design, construction, and testing of protective eyewear. The eyewear standards include the following minimum requirements: protective eyewear must protect against the hazards for which they were designed and be reasonably comfortable to allow prolonged use but fit securely without interfering with movement or vision. The standards mandate that the eyewear be capable of disinfection and be easily cleansable. Only eyewear that has been tested and shown to prevent against pathogen transmission and offer impact resistance may be marked "Z87" meaning that the construction meets Z87.1-1979 standards [16]. Secondary protectors, including face shields, may be used as an adjunct to the use of protective eyewear. OSHA regulations mandate that primary ANSI Z87.1 eye protection "must be provided to all employees." OSHA standards also require that employers ensure that "each affected employee uses appropriate eye or face protection when exposed to hazards" [17]. The hazards outlined include airborne particles, projectiles, vapors, and harmful light. When a wearer of protective eyewear must use prescription lenses, OSHA requires that the provided eyewear incorporate the prescription lenses into the design or allow for wearing the prescription lenses under the eyewear.

Blood-borne pathogens

More than 200 different diseases may be transmitted from exposure to blood. Three of the most serious in terms of long-term health risks are hepatitis B virus (HBV), hepatitis C virus (HCV), and HIV. Although the risks are low from any one exposure, oral surgeons and dentists frequently are working in an intra- or extraoral field where patient blood is present. Exposure to pathogens occurs when a health care provider comes into contact with blood or a bloody fluid, such as serosanguineous fluid, phlegm, or urine, containing blood or another bodily fluid. Disease transmission occurs only if the bodily fluid containing pathogens comes into contact with a part of the body through which absorption can take place. Fluids containing viruses, such as coolant spray from a surgical handpiece that has mixed with blood, must come into contact with mucous membranes of the eye or mouth for transmission to occur. Pathogen-containing fluid also may be transmitted through exposure to skin that is not intact, such as skin with cuts, scrapes, or rashes or through thin skin membranes of the genitals. Any exposure to a large amount of blood or exposure to a large surface area of intact skin constitutes a transmission risk. There are other factors that influence risk, such as the quantity of blood or fluid exposure and the depth and size of a penetrating injury. The viral load of the infections blood also may affect this risk. Prospective studies that examined health care workers who had mucous membrane exposure to HIV showed no conversion among those exposed. There are cases, however, where no other explanation has been found for health care workers who contracted HIV and mucous membrane exposure is believed the only source of transmission. The risk for acquiring HIV thus is believed to be less than 0.3%.

Among the most easily transmitted viruses is HBV. A health care worker who sustains a needlestick with blood from a known HBV-infected patient has a 6% to 30% chance of contracting HBV. In the same situation, the risk for HCV infection is 1.8% and for HIV is less than 0.3% [18]. Fortunately, there now is an effective HBV vaccine formulated from proteins and not HBV itself. If workers have not had prophylactic vaccination with the HBV vaccine, the vaccine should be given as soon as possible after the exposure and at 1- and 6-month intervals after the exposure. Hepatitis B immune globulin containing antibodies to HBV also should be given at the time of exposure and the first dose of HBV vaccine. HCV is transmitted less easily but there are no known effective means for preventing infection after an exposure. Blood tests after an exposure should be performed to determine if transmission and conversion have occurred. Subsequent liver tests should be performed if symptoms of loss of appetite, nausea, abdominal pain, darkening of urine, light stools, or jaundice develop after an exposure.

Microscopic blood- and fluid-borne pathogens

The most frequently requested information from OSHA is on management of risks associated with blood and other bodily fluid–borne pathogens. Blood-borne pathogens are micro-organisms present in human blood that may cause harm to humans. HBV and HIV are two examples of pathogens that oral health care professionals are at risk for exposure to when in contact with patients. In 1992, an OSHA Bloodborne Pathogens Standard took effect with the aim of preventing more than 200 deaths and 9000 blood-borne infections [19]. The standard is aimed primarily at clinics and hospitals and all other places where workers might be exposed to blood and other potentially infectious materials. The purpose of the standard is to limit exposure to blood, saliva, and other infectious materials that could lead to the transmission of blood-borne pathogens causing disease or death.

The rules for prevention of transmission of blood- and fluid-borne pathogens are straightforward and lifesaving in the health care workplace. OSHA regulations state that eating, drinking, or applying lip balms or handling contact lenses should be avoided in areas where occupational exposure may occur. Areas where direct patient contact takes place are an example of OSHA restricted areas for eating and drinking or application of cosmetics or products to protect the lips. Placing or repositioning contact lenses should be avoided in direct patient contact areas. The Bloodborne Pathogens Standard contains a Good Samaritan clause so that acts, such as "assisting a co-worker with a nosebleed would not be considered occupational exposure" [20]. Potentially infectious materials identified in the standard include blood, saliva, and all other body fluids, including cerebrospinal fluid and pleural fluid. OSHA blood-borne pathogens standards also govern the use of graft materials, including any unfixed tissue or organ other than intact skin from a human living donor or cadaver.

The OSHA blood-borne pathogen standards require employers to have written guidelines in place for the management of an occupation exposure to potentially infectious materials. To comply with the standards, universal precautions must be in place. Under universal precautions, all body fluids, including blood and tissue, are considered potentially infectious. Thus, handwashing before and after all patient encounters is part of the standard of care. Employers must provide facilities and ensure that employees use them before and after patient contact. Other requirements of employers in the blood-borne pathogens standards include an annual exposure control plan; use of new technologies that reduce the risk for needlesticks, such as self-capping needles; and use of labeled and color-coded specimen and regulated waste containers.

Needlestick and other sharps injuries

The Needlestick Prevention and Safety Act was passed by Congress in 2000 and required that OSHA update and revise safety standards with regard to needlesticks. In response to this act, in 2001, OSHA updated standards of the blood-borne pathogens section of the safety code. Employers now are required to provide new needles and devices that minimize needlestick exposures as they become available. Studies over the past few years indicate that approximately 600,000 to 800,000 needlestick injuries occur annually to health care workers [21]. Newer, self-protective needle capping syringes are one example. The code mandates that employees be given the opportunity to review and help select needlestick prevention devices. In addition, as part of the updated code, employers are responsible for maintaining a log of needlestick exposures. The intention of the log is to help in the annual review so that workplace protocol may be modified to reduce the number of exposures. The OSHA code requires that all logs of needlestick incidents protect the privacy of employees. Employers must provide personal protective equipment, including gloves, gowns, and masks, to prevent potential pathogen exposure. The act specifies methods for disposing contaminated sharps and sets forth standards for containers for these items and other regulated waste. Studies suggest that one third of needlesticks occur during attempted disposal of needles [22].

OSHA requires that a process be in place if an exposure incident should occur. Any laboratory tests that are indicated must be conducted by an accredited laboratory at no cost to employees. A confidential medical examination post exposure must be conducted in which the circumstances of exposure are recorded. Testing must be performed provided that the source individual agrees. Postexposure prophylaxis and counseling and evaluation of reported illnesses must be performed. The hepatitis B vaccine must be supplied by an employer within 10 working days of a new employee's hire. The vaccine must be provided at no cost. No provisions or prescreening may be required by an employer to obtain the vaccine. Employees may choose not to be vaccinated at the time of initial employment; therefore, they may choose to receive a hepatitis B vaccination or booster at any time during employment. At that time, the employers must offer the vaccine [23].

Housekeeping

All equipment and environmental and work surfaces must be cleaned and decontaminated after contact with blood or other infectious materials. All potentially contaminated work surfaces must be cleaned with an appropriate cleanser before and after concluding patient visits. Any overtly contaminated surface must be cleaned as soon as possible. Appropriate solutions for cleaning include diluted bleach solution and Environmental Protection Agency–registered tuberculocides and cleansers known to eradicate HBV/HIV. The Environmental Protection Agency Web site [24] lists registered approved cleansers. Protective coverings that cannot be cleaned must be removed and replaced. Frequent inspection of all disposal containers is mandatory each day and cleaning and decontamination of these receptacles must occur on a regular basis. Should a spill occur of blood or other potentially infectious fluid, it must be soaked up and the area decontaminated immediately. All employees involved in preparing patient care workspaces must wear gloves when decontaminating instruments and work surfaces.

Sharps containers and regulated waste disposal

Needles and sharp instruments are a potential source of injury in the dental office. OSHA regulations govern work practice controls for needle handling. In 2001, revisions to OSHA's Bloodborne Pathogens Standard as mandated by the Needlestick Safety and Prevention Act of 2000 went into effect. These revisions mandated that all employers consider safer needle protection devices, such as self-capping needles, as they become available. OSHA regulations apply only to use and disposal of sharps and medical waste within dental offices. Once disposed material is taken out of an office, OSHA has no authority over its disposal. Recent changes exempt all dental practices from keeping a separate sharps injury log. The only rare exception is when OSHA or the Bureau of Labor Statistics requires maintenance of logs as part of national data gathering on workplace injuries and illnesses. OSHA Forms 300 and 301 may be used for this purpose in this rare case.

Amalgam waste disposal

Dental amalgam is comprised of a combination of mercury and an alloy consisting of silver, tin copper, zinc, and other trace metals. The potential for incorrect disposal of amalgam containing mercury in the public water supply is a concern of environmental groups. All mercury-containing products, including dental amalgam, is regulated by acts of Congress, including the Clean Water Act; the Environmental Protection Agency; and other state and local environmental agencies. Alternatively, dental organizations argue that because dental mercury is bound up in the solid form of amalgam, its disposal has little impact on the environment. There has never been scientific proof of harm caused by dental amalgam on the environment [25]. Because dental amalgam is identified as a potential source of environmental harm, however, specific guidelines exist regarding the safe handling and management of amalgam in dental offices.

The first regulator to contact a dental office often is a publicly owned wastewater treatment plant. These facilities have limits for mercury that are set by the state. The treatment plants are required to meet these limits and to reduce mercury discharge. All industries, businesses, and dental offices are contacted initially if the target limit is not met. The authority of the waste management plants is wide ranging; penalty fines initially may be imposed leading up to a total ban on mercury containing product use. The relationship of water treatment facilities with dental offices most often is cooperative, encouraging dental offices to dispose of amalgam in separate containers and to use amalgam separators if necessary. The ADA has published recommendations and guidelines for amalgam management in dental offices, published under the heading of best management practices. Developed in 2006, the ANSI and the ADA developed specifications describing the procedures for storing and preparing amalgam waste for delivery to recyclers (ANSA/ADA Specification 109). The specific containers for storing and shipping amalgam are described in Specification 109. Containers for amalgam waste must have a silver or gray label and must be marked "Amalgam Waste for Recycling." Containers must have a sealable closure and must meet requirements set by the Department of Transportation and the International Safe Transportation Association. Some cities and states have regulations regarding amalgam waste handling that are more strict and require dental practices to install amalgam separators. The ADA has published information regarding the use of amalgam separators, and state and local dental societies may have recommendations regarding their state specific laws for amalgam handling.

Material Safety Data Sheets

Material Safety Data Sheets (MSDS) list the specific information on the chemicals used in an operatory and office. MSDS offer detailed information bulletins prepared by the manufacturer or supplier of any product that contains a chemical deemed hazardous. The physical and chemical properties and any potentially hazardous properties, such as flammability or combustibility, are described. Health hazards associated with the use of the chemicals, routes of exposure, and precautions for safe handling are included in MSDS. Each MSDS should contain a section on the control of exposure to the chemical used and first-aid measures that may be taken in the case of an emergent spill or leak. An office employer and manager must maintain a file of MSDS supplied by manufacturers or suppliers. Acquiring, filing, and updating MSDS regularly are the responsibility of the employer and manager of an office. Manufacturers of products and chemicals used should be contacted if additional information is needed or to obtain MSDS. Furthermore, a master list of all chemicals and an index of the location of MSDS must be accessible to all employees.

Vaccinations

Vaccinations must be made available to all employees who have occupational exposure to blood within 10 working days of assignment, at no cost, at a reasonable time and place, under the supervision of licensed physician/licensed health care professional, and according to the latest recommendations of the United States Public Health Service. Prescreening may not be required as a condition of receiving a vaccine. Employees must sign a declination form if they choose not to be vaccinated but later may opt to receive a vaccine at no cost to the employee. Should booster doses later be recommended by the Public Health Service, employees must be offered updated vaccinations.

Hazard communication

Required warning labels include the orange or orange-red biohazard symbol affixed to containers of regulated waste, refrigerators and freezers, and other containers used to store or transport blood or other potentially infectious materials. Red bags or containers may be used instead of labeling. When a facility uses universal precautions in its handling of all specimens, labeling is not required within the facility. Likewise, when all laundry is handled with universal precautions, the laundry need not be labeled. Blood that has been tested and found free of HIV or HBV and released for clinical use and regulated waste that has been decontaminated need not be labeled. Signs must be used to identify restricted areas in HIV and HBV research laboratories and production facilities.

Information and training

Mandated training is required within 90 days of the start date, initially on assignment and annually—employees who have received appropriate training within the past year need only receive additional training in items not previously covered. Training must include making accessible a copy of the regulatory text of a standard and explanation of its contents, general discussion on blood-borne diseases and their transmission, exposure control plan, engineering and work practice controls, personal protective equipment, hepatitis B vaccine, response to emergencies involving blood, how to handle exposure incidents, postexposure evaluation and follow-up program, and signs/labels/color coding. There must be opportunity for questions and answers, and trainers must be knowledgeable in the subject matter. Laboratory and production facility workers must receive additional specialized initial training.

Record keeping

OSHA requires that documentation of training sessions and medical records be kept up to date. Full compliance with OSHA standards requires documentation, when a new employee is hired, of the new employee's "occupational exposure" risk to blood-borne pathogens. Confidential medical records must be kept for employees, including employee name, social security number, and hepatitis B vaccination status. Employees must be informed of their right to access personal medical records. The level of training for dental practice workplace injury risks must be assessed and additional training must be offered depending on the specific risks present in an office. Training in the prevention of risks present in the dental office, such as exposure to blood-borne pathogens and sharps injuries, must be given to all new employees. Furthermore, when a dental employee takes on a new responsibility, relevant training in reduction of risk exposure must be documented.

Medical records must be kept for each employee who is at risk for occupational exposure to hazardous chemicals or materials for the duration of a worker's employment plus 30 years [26]. These records must be confidential and must include employee name and social security number; hepatitis B vaccination status (including dates); results of any examinations, medical testing, and follow-up procedures; a copy of the health care professional's written opinion; and a copy of information provided to the health care professional. Training records must be maintained for 3 years and must include dates, contents of the training program or a summary, trainer's name and qualifications, and names and job titles of all persons attending the sessions. Medical records must be made available to the subject employee, anyone who has written consent from the employee, OSHA, and NIOSH—they are not available to an employer. Disposal of records must be in accord with OSHA's standard covering access to records.

Reporting injuries in the dental office

Dental offices are exempt from federal OSHA requirements for routine maintenance of a log of injuries and illnesses. A dental office may be required to keep logs of staff injuries and illnesses only if requested in advance by the Bureau of Labor Statistics. OSHA Form 300 may be used for the purpose of providing data on injuries in a dental office. OSHA Form 300 is available at http://www.osha.gov/recordkeeping/new-osha300form1-1-04.pdf. Fatal injuries or dental clinic injuries resulting in a hospitalization of at least three employees must be reported to OSHA within 8 hours. The dentist in charge of a practice must report a fatality or multiple hospitalizations by telephone or in person to the OSHA area office nearest the site of the incident. The toll-free central OSHA telephone number (listed previously) also may be used to report serious injuries. OSHA requires dentists to maintain a confidential medical record for each employee who may be exposed to blood-borne pathogens and other potentially infectious materials. Medical records for employees must be retained according to OSHA regulations for an employee's period of employment plus 30 years. When a practice is sold or ownership is transferred, the records of all former and current employees must be transferred to the new practice owner or the NIOSH if there is no new owner. All medical records must be available to employees of a dental practice and to OSHA inspectors who have authorized access. Legally, the owner of a dental practice may request a subpoena in such cases from an OSHA inspector before release of medical records. The head of a dental practice must keep a copy on file of OSHA's Access to Medical Records Standard.

Maintaining a safe clinic environment and equipment

The physical premises of practice offices must meet OSHA workplace safety standards. To protect against fire, an automatic sprinkler system must be maintained in reliable operating condition at all times. Practice owners should maintain a fire emergency plan and inform all employees of the planned action in the event of a fire. For larger practices, this plan must be given to employees in written form. Portable fire extinguishers must be kept accessible in offices and clinics. OSHA requires the maintenance of extinguishers and mandates training for all employees in the use of extinguishers unless a fire safety plan calls for immediate evacuation of all employees. Portable fire extinguishers must be checked annually and records kept for each annual maintenance check. A first-aid kit and at least one person trained to render aid and administer basic life support are requirements for all general practice offices located outside of a town where a clinic or hospital is present. Sufficient exits must be present to allow for immediate escape during an emergency. The construction of an office must not place the lives and safety of occupants in danger. Exit signs must be marked clearly and exit doors must not be locked during hours when dentists or staff are at work in the office. All other doors that might be mistaken for exit doors during an emergency must have clear signs indicating "closet" or "supply room" to reduce the risk for confusion during an emergency. OSHA requires that all compressed gas tanks that are used be kept in good condition and that they be sufficiently secured to prevent tipping. All such gas cylinders must be checked on a regular basis to ensure they are intact. In the event of an exposure, quick flush and eyewash facilities must be available. Such eyewash stations may be purchased through safety catalogs. Waste must be disposed of in containers that have covers. The containers should be resistant to corrosion and easily cleanable. These containers should not be overfilled. If the space where a general practice office is located is leased, all communication regarding safety concerns with the building owner must be retained and submitted to an OSHA inspector on an OSHA site visit.

Inspections and postinspection procedures

OSHA inspectors conduct site visits with the intent of calling attention to any unsafe working conditions or practices. Warrants before all visits by OSHA inspectors and subpoenas before any release of medical records may be requested by a dentist under investigation. A dentist under investigation is not obligated to agree with any assertions by an OSHA inspector. Any such agreements may be taken as an admission against the interest of a dentist in charge of a practice. A practice owner should not admit to any violations and should take the inspector's recommendations under advisement. An OSHA inspection may not interfere with patient care and should a disagreement occur regarding the interruption of patient care privacy, the general practice dentist should consult an attorney. Should a complaint be presented as the initial reason for an OSHA inspection, the complaint should be reviewed carefully before the inspection begins. The practice owner should ask the inspector what specific areas are planned for inspection. The owner of a practice has the right to be present during an inspection. Employers in dental practices are held responsible for all employee OSHA violations. If an employer fails to enforce employees to maintain proper hand hygiene and wear gloves during patient encounters, for example, the employer may be cited.

During an inspection, evidence is gathered by the OSHA inspectors to support citations and penalties. Evidence may include copies of records, photographs of the work environment, and statements made by a practice owner or employees of a practice. Employees are not required to speak with an inspector but they may not be inhibited from making statements to an inspector. An inspector may request to interview employees without a practice owner or manager present. Any false statements given to an OSHA inspector are a violation of the law. All citations for the practice must be provided to employees in written form. After any citations, a practice owner has 15 working days to contest the citations. An informal hearing with OSHA regulators follows and a reduction in fines or, less frequently, a retraction of the citation may be granted. The 15 working day period may not be extended for any reason. Legal counsel is advised when contesting OSHA citations. The contesting of a citation follows a specific legal format beginning with, "On behalf of [empoyer's name], I hereby contest the citation[s] issued, each item in the citation[s], the proposed penalties, the proposed abatement and abatement dates and all matters subject to protest." The violation cited during an OSHA inspection must be corrected as soon as possible and failure to do so may result in additional fines.

Occupational Safety and Health Administration helpline

OSHA has a helpline that was established in 1991. The telephone number, (800) 321-OSHA (6742), provides access to an automated system that answers many common OSHA-related questions. Requests for current print publications also may be made through the helpline.

Summary

OSHA became part of the United States Department of Labor in 1971. The aim of OSHA is to regulate the workplaces for workers in the dental profession in an attempt to ensure safety. OSHA protects health care workers from injury at the workplace by providing suggestions from better ergonomics to inspecting health care facilities to ensure proper sterilization procedures. OSHA has a record of success in the endeavor of workplace safety. Since it was formed in 1971, fatalities at work in all sectors have been reduced by 60%. Illnesses and injury have been reduced by 40% [27]. OSHA has more than 2000 employees, including more than 1000 inspectors. There are OSHA offices in all 50 states. The current administration's mandate for OSHA is to enforce the standards for workplace safety, to communicate workplace health and safety standards to employers and workers, and to partner with other programs to promote workplace safety.

References

[1] U.S. Department of Labor, Bureau of Labor Statistics. Injuries, illness and fatalities. Census of fatal workplace injuries 1992–2002. Available at: www.bls.gov. Accessed February 2, 2008.

[2] Occupational Safety and Health Administration. Available at: http://www.osha.gov/dcsp/compliance_assistance/quickstarts/health_care/healthcare/health_care.html.

[3] U.S. Department of Labor, Bureau of Labor Statistics. Injuries, illness and fatalities. Census of fatal workplace injuries 2006. Available at: www.bls.gov. Accessed February 2, 2008.
[4] Weinberg K. Surviving OSHA: how to avoid, manage, and respond to healthcare inspections. Hcpro; 2004.
[5] OSHA bloodborne pathogen standard, 29 CFR 1910.1030, U.S. Department of Labor Fact Sheet No. OSHA 92–46. Available at: http://www.osha.gov/publications/OSHA3187/osha3187.html.
[6] OSHA bloodborne pathogen standard, 1910.1030(d)(2)(vi), U.S. Department of Labor Fact Sheet No. OSHA 92–50. Available at: http://www.osha.gov/publications.
[7] OSHA regulations and Standards—29 CFR, eye and face protection 1910.33. Available at: http://www.osha.gov/publications/OSHA3187/osha3187.html.
[8] Gerberding JL. Management of occupational exposures to blood-borne viruses. N Engl J Med 1995;332:444.
[9] Makary MA, Al-Attar A, Holzmueller CG, et al. Needlestick injuries are common but unreported by surgeons in training. N Engl J Med 2007;356:2693.
[10] OSHA national news release, US Department of Labor; Office of Public Affairs. Needlestick requirements take effect April 18, 2001.
[11] Selecting, evaluating, and using sharps disposal containers. U.S. Department of Health and Human Services, Public Health Service, Centers for Disease Control and Prevention, National Institute for Occupational Safety and Health, Atlanta, Georgia, January 1998 DHHS (NIOSH) publication No 97–111. Available at: http://www.cdc.gov/niosh/sharps1.html.
[12] McDonald LL. The influence of the Occupational Safety and Health Administration on infection control practice. nursing clinics of North America 1993;28(3):613–24.
[13] Hazard Communication Standard (29 CFR 1910.1200). Available at: http://www.osha-slc.gov/OshStd. Accessed February 2, 2008.
[14] Bernstein JA. Material safety data sheets: are they reliable in identifying human hazards? J Allergy Clin Immunol 2002;110:35–8.
[15] Fishman MC, Triadafilopoulos G, et al. Medicine. 5th edition. Philadelphia: Lippincott, Williams & Wilkins; 2004.
[16] Harrison's medical manual of medicine. 15th edition. New York: McGraw Hill; 2002.
[17] Centers for Disease Control and Prevention. Revised classification system for HIV infection and expanded case surveillance definition for AIDS among adolescents and adults. MMWR Recomm Rep 1992;41(RR-17):1–19.
[18] Gerson RR, Karkashian C, Felnor S. Universal precautions: an update. Heart Lung 1994; 23(4):352–8.
[19] McCunney RJ. Medical surveillance: the role of the family physician. Am Fam Physician 2001;63(12):2339–40.
[20] Pepys J, Berstein IL. Historical aspects of occupational asthma. In: Berstein IL, Chan-Yeung M, Malo JL, et al, editors. Asthma in the workplace. 2nd edition. New York: Marcel Dekker, Inc.; 1999. p. 5–26.
[21] Beckett WS. Occupational respiratory diseases. N Engl J Med 2000;342:406–13.
[22] Gerson RR. Barriers to precaution adoption among health care workers [thesis]. Baltimore (MD): JKohns Hopkins University; 1990.
[23] Marcus R. The Centers for Disease Control Cooperative Needlestick Surveillance Group. Surveillance of health care workers exposed to blood from patients infected with the human immunodeficiency virus. N Engl J Med 1988;319:1118–23.
[24] Environmental Protection Agency. Available at: http://www.epa.gov.
[25] Mangione CM, Gerberding JL, Cummings SR. Occupational exposure to HIV: frequency and rates of underreporting of percutaneous and mucocutaneous exposures by housestaff. Am J Med 1991;90:85–90.
[26] Hamory B. Underreporting of needlestick injuries in a university hospital. Am J Infect Control 1983;11:174–7.
[27] Jagger J, Hurt EH, Brand-Elnaggar J, et al. Rates of needlestick injury caused by various devices in a university hospital. N Engl J Med 1988;319:284–8.

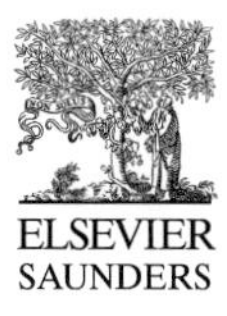

ELSEVIER
SAUNDERS

THE DENTAL CLINICS OF NORTH AMERICA

Dent Clin N Am 52 (2008) 669–682

How to Implement a HIPAA Compliance Plan into a Practice

Edmund Wun, DDS[a], Harry Dym, DDS[b,c,d,*]

[a]*Department of Dentistry and Oral and Maxillofacial Surgery, The Brooklyn Hospital Center, 121 Dekalb Avenue, Brooklyn, NY 11201, USA*

[b]*Department of Dentistry and Oral Maxillofacial Surgery, The Brooklyn Hospital Center, 121 Dekalb Avenue, Brooklyn, NY 11201, USA*

[c]*Woodhull Medical Hospital, Brooklyn, NY, USA*

[d]*Department of Oral and Maxillofacial Surgery, Columbia University College of Dental Medicine, New York, NY, USA*

For a practice to succeed today, practitioners must look toward their patients' well-being in the office setting and outside as well. In the office setting, such care includes a thorough patient history as well as an impeccable clinical examination. Outside the office setting, the practitioner must safeguard the patient from a different type of threat—the invasion of privacy. Every patient has the right to privacy and security of his or her personal information. For this reason, the Health Insurance Portability and Accountability Act (HIPAA) of 1996 was created. How does a practitioner ensure that his or her practice is compliant and that patient information is truly kept private? This article addresses these concerns and explores what a practice should include and undergo to ultimately become HIPAA compliant to better protect the patient in the office and out.

The Department of Health and Human Services has been given the responsibility of creating regulations to help practices become HIPAA compliant. These regulations may be divided into three main categories: the Standards for Electronic Transactions, the Security and Electronic Signature Standards, and the Standards for Privacy of Individually Identifiable Health Information (IIHI). By following these three regulations, a practice should be able to reduce the cost to become HIPAA compliant as well as simplify the process.

The information herein has been summarized and condensed from McGraw S, Plotzker S. Health Insurance Portability and Accountability Act (HIPAA) Compliance Plan. Plymouth Meeting (PA): The Health Care Group; 2002. Available at: http://www.healthcaregroup.com.

* Corresponding author. Department of Dentistry and Oral Maxillofacial Surgery, The Brooklyn Hospital Center, 121 Dekalb Avenue, Brooklyn, NY 11201.

E-mail address: hdymdds@yahoo.com (H. Dym).

0011-8532/08/$ - see front matter
doi:10.1016/j.cden.2008.02.006 ***dental.theclinics.com***

The Standards for Electronic Transactions oversee eight specific electronic transactions: (1) health care claims encounter information, (2) eligibility for a health plan, (3) referral certification and authorization, (4) health care claim status, (5) enrollment and disenrollment in a health plan, (6) health care payment and remittance advice, (7) health care premium payments, and (8) coordination of benefits. The fact that these transactions are electronic requires a practice's current technology to be compliant; therefore, practitioners should contact their software vendors to confirm that their software is indeed HIPAA compliant. Also included in these standards is a specific code set for electronic transactions regarding health care, including Current Procedural Terminology-4 (CPT-4) codes, ICD-9-CM (International Classification of Diseases, 9th revision, clinical modification) diagnosis codes, Health Care Financing Administration Common Procedural Coding System (HCPCS) equipment and supply codes, and National Drug Codes (NDC). For those practitioners exposed to mental health disorders, Diagnostic and Statistical Manual IV (DSM IV) codes are not accepted.

The Security and Electronic Signature Standards have been put in place to prevent unauthorized parties from accessing protected health information (PHI). Examples of these standards are the requirement of a practice's information technology systems to include firewalls, mechanisms to authenticate both the identity and E-mail address of anyone sending information, procedures to recover lost data, and staff limitations to access of information.

The Standards for Privacy of IIHI are an essential component of the regulations. They require that a covered entity (including health care providers transmitting health information in electronic form, private and federally funded insurers, and health care clearinghouses) create policy and procedure regulations to safeguard individually identifiable health information as well as those that come into contact with this information. An effective policy will enforce these guidelines as well as educate and notify employees and contractors.

Practitioners should be aware that a HIPAA compliance plan should be custom-made to fit their practice, but each plan should also contain the basic elements that have been included within the regulations. Depending on the offense, fines for the failure to comply with HIPAA regulations can range from $100 per person per violation to $250,000 with or without imprisonment of not more than 10 years. The HIPAA regulations preempt all state regulations unless it is determined that state law provides stricter protection of patients' PHI.

HIPAA plan requirements

Before delving into the specifics of the HIPAA compliance plan, it is important to realize what basic elements should be covered within. A practitioner's HIPAA compliance plan should discuss the following:

Privacy officer—appointed to oversee HIPAA privacy compliance efforts

Security officer—appointed to oversee HIPAA information systems security compliance efforts (may be same person as above and titled "compliance officer for HIPAA privacy and security")
An HIPAA compliance committee chaired by above officers (compliance personnel)—should represent practitioners as well as staff from front desk, billing, nursing, and medical records
Baseline audit of current procedures and determination of potential or current leaks of PHI
Development and implementation of plan for maintaining privacy—should include written standards, policies, and procedures
Development of open lines of communication—should include, but not be limited to, the following: adding HIPAA issues to staff meeting agendas, updates regarding practice HIPAA compliance activities, and so on
Regular staff training/education to cover practice standards and procedures
Establishment and use of written agreements with business associates
Development and posting of a "notice of privacy practices"
Development of forms for consent and authorization
Detection of current violations and investigation of any allegations, followed by disclosure of incidents to proper government entities
System for reporting complaints
Enforcing publicized disciplinary standards
The practice's own specific needs

It is expected that the needs of an individual practice will differ from that of another and will also change as time passes; therefore, it is important to continually update the practice's compliance needs and identify and address potential areas of risk and exposure of information.

Key terms

HIPAA uses the following terminology in their legislation:

Business associate—a person/entity acting on behalf of a covered entity (not as an employee) to assist in any function involving actual/potential disclosure of IIHI (ie, independent contractor providers [eg, physicians, dentists, contract managers, billing services], accountants, lawyers, software vendors, and any person/entity that does business with a covered entity when IIHI can be exchanged or disclosed)
Covered entity—any person/organization that transmits (or has a business associate who transmits on their behalf) any IIHI, whether in an electronic format or not (eg, health plans, health care clearinghouses, health care providers)
Health care provider—includes physicians and dentists and their respective practices, hospitals, skilled nursing facilities, comprehensive outpatient rehabilitation facilities, home health agencies, hospices, and those

providing any medical, dental, nursing, or allied health services; health care providers transmitting health information in electronic format considered covered entities, with privacy regulations applying to electronic and non-electronic information

Health information—any information created/received by a health care provider that relates to (1) the past, present, or future health condition of an individual; (2) the provision of health care to an individual; or (3) the past, present, or future payment for provision of health care; includes anything transmitted or recorded in any medium (eg, orally, electronically, by tape)

IIHI—any information that (1) is created/received by a health care provider, health plan, employer, or health care clearinghouse; (2) relates to the past, present, or future physical/mental health or condition of an individual, including the past, present, or future payment for provision of health care to an individual; (3) may actually or reasonably identify an individual; includes, but is not limited to, demographic information, patient name, address, E-mail, phone/fax numbers, social security numbers

PHI—IIHI that can be associated with an individual and transmitted/maintained electronically or in another medium, such as benefit management information, claims/encounter forms, claim status information, coordination of benefits or information, eligibility for a health plan, explanations of benefits, reports of injury, health claim attachments, health data analysis (specific to individuals, not the practice), payment/remittance forms, referral forms, or other transactions as may be prescribed by regulation

Applicability and standards for protected health information

General standards

The advancement of technology continually creates new opportunities for the potential compromise of the integrity and confidentiality of PHI. Providers are responsible for how PHI is, and could potentially be, used by others, including business associates; therefore, they are required to terminate business relations with those who inappropriately use it. Otherwise, the Department of Health and Human Services should be contacted. Only the minimum amount of information necessary for the task should be released.

Federal regulations allow patients the right to inspect, copy, or request changes to their medical records. Dentists and physicians require permission to share patient information for billing and treatment purposes, and health care providers must disclose how this information will be used and disclose only the minimum information necessary to accomplish these tasks. HIPAA compliance agreements must exist between covered entities and business partners, and appropriate business practices must exist within these organizations. Otherwise, criminal or civil penalties may result.

Notice of privacy practices

A written notice of the practice's policies and procedures regarding the use and disclosure of PHI must be provided for the patient, including the patient's rights and the practice's legal duties. This notice must be clear and include the following:

- A description of how PHI may be disclosed (including treatment, payment, health care operations) with at least one example
- A description of instances in which the provider may use/disclose PHI without the patient's consent/authorization
- Provisions of state law, if more stringent
- A statement that authorization must be obtained for any other uses
- A description of the patient's right to access, inspect, copy, and amend their own records, including the procedure to do so
- A description of the patient's right to request restrictions on the provider's policies as contained in the notice and the procedure to do so
- A description of the patient's right to receive an accounting of any disclosures
- A description of the patient's right to receive a paper copy of the notice
- A procedure for filing a complaint with the practice and the Department of Health and Human Services if it is believed that privacy rights have been violated
- A statement that the practice is required by law to protect PHI and is bound by terms of the notice
- If applicable, a statement that the practice may contact the patient for appointment reminders or to transmit relevant information about treatment alternatives

The notice of privacy practices must be clearly visible in a prominent location, and paper copies of the notice must be given to patients upon request. Practice Web sites also must have the notice on prominent display. If the notice is lengthy, a summary may be provided in addition to the notice, not instead. The summary should be one or two pages in length with the notice underneath it. This combination is called a "layered notice."

Consent versus authorization

A written acknowledgment of a patient's receipt of the notice or authorization must be obtained. If the PHI is to be used for treatment, payment, or health care operations (TPO), only a written acknowledgment is required. All other uses (eg, research, fundraising, marketing) require a more specific authorization.

Written acknowledgment/consent

If PHI is to be used for TPO purposes only, the patient must sign a written acknowledgment that he or she has received the notice. If the patient refuses, the attempt must be documented. The patient's PHI may still be used for TPO purposes. Currently, there is no prescribed form for the written acknowledgment; a consent may be used instead. Consents should be separate from the notice, written in plain language, and include the following:

- A statement that PHI may be used for any of the TPO purposes
- Reference to the notice while providing patients the chance to review it
- Reservation of the right to change the practice's privacy policies and how the patient may be notified
- The right of patients to restrict PHI use beyond the practice's policies, with a statement that the practice does not have to agree to additional restrictions; should the practice agree, the patient's additional limitations become binding
- A statement that the patient may revoke the consent in writing at any time
- The patient's signature and date

Authorizations and accounting

Typical authorizations involve disclosures for research, marketing, or fundraising. The practice may not condition any provision of health care based on these authorizations. Authorizations must include the following:

- A specific description of the information to be used or disclosed
- The identification of specific individuals who may use/disclose the information as well as those who may receive and use the disclosed information
- A description of each purpose of requested use or disclosure
- The expiration date of the use or disclosure
- A statement of the patient's right to revoke the authorization in writing at any time along with the procedure to do so
- A statement that the PHI used/disclosed may be subject to redisclosure by the receiving party and may no longer be protected
- The patient's signature and date

A separate authorization must be completed for each use or disclosure. An account must be recorded of all non-TPO use of PHI for 6 years. This accounting must be provided at any time per the patient's request.

When authorization is not required

PHI may be released without authorization in the following situations:

- If the information is used for TPO purposes, for a marketing communication that is face-to-face, or a promotional gift of nominal value
- For research purposes when an authorization is independently approved by a privacy board or institutional review board
- In judicial/administrative proceedings, in limited law enforcement activities, or in investigations of abuse/neglect

For identification of a deceased person or cause of death
For activities related to national defense

Authorization is also not required for health care information with no individually identifiable information.

Opportunity to agree or object situation

A patient's verbal consent, agreement, or objection to the use or disclosure of PHI may be permitted as long as the patient is informed of how it will be used. Another instance includes hospital verification of admittance and the provision of a room number or the general condition of a patient. Failure to object in this case will also suffice.

Patient access to information

At all times, a patient may view, request a copy of, amend, or receive a list of those entities that have seen their medical information within the past 6 years. Upon a reasonable request to do so, the practice will honor this obligation, unless the practice feels that doing so will endanger the life or physical safety of said individual. Generally, providers have 30 days from the request date to provide the appropriate information. A summary may suffice and a reasonable fee may be charged as well. There is no requirement to provide data from another provider or that which is believed to be inaccurate.

Special issues related to psychotherapy notes

Under extremely limited exceptions, specific authorizations are always required for the use or disclosure of psychotherapy notes.

Research

Unless the research is included under the waiver of authorization provisions including medical treatment, approval of valid waivers of authorization must be obtained by a provider, by an institutional review board established in accordance with applicable federal law, or by a privacy board comprised of members with varied backgrounds and appropriate professional competencies including at least one member. To obtain approval, the research must not be able to be completed without the PHI. There must also be limited risk of loss of privacy, and it must be shown that it is not practicable to perform the research unless a waiver is granted.

De-identification and re-identification

De-identified information is no longer PHI, that is, it is not subject to the privacy regulations, whereas re-identified information becomes PHI and is subject to the rules. PHI may be de-identified in one of two ways. First, a covered entity may use a person or entity with appropriate knowledge or experience of the generally accepted statistical and scientific principles or methods for rendering information not individually identifiable. The same is true for those anticipating receipt of said information. Second, any identifiers of the individual or the relatives, employers, or household members of the individual may be removed from the data by the covered entity. A method of re-identifying the information may be assigned by the covered entity as long as certain security criteria are met.

Minimum necessary rule

The minimum amount of PHI necessary to accomplish a certain task must be disclosed. Situations in which covered entities are not required to make a minimum necessary determination are as follows:

When the disclosure is made to/requested by a health care provider for treatment
When the uses/disclosures are made to the individual who is the subject of PHI
When the subject of PHI requests accounting of disclosures of PHI
When the disclosure of PHI is requested by the Secretary of Health and Human Services to determine the covered entity's compliance with the rule, or is required from compliance with applicable requirements of the rule
When the use/disclosure is required by law and the use/disclosure complies with, and is limited to, the relevant requirements of such law

Staff training

All staff must be educated in the practice's privacy and security policies and procedures and must be notified of policy and procedure changes, as well as changes in the law. New employees must be trained shortly after employment begins.

Security concerns

Practices need to be able to verify the recipients of PHI that is sent. They also need to authenticate the source of any PHI that is received, and they must be able to encode information to prevent unintended interceptions of PHI. Security of the system from outsiders using firewalls and the like is mandatory. Covered entities should also create chain of trust agreements with whomever the PHI is exchanged, requiring those contacting the practice's PHI to be bound by the same security requirements as the practice. Computers should be in private secure locations and should have a secure password to limit access to the computer and potential PHI. Practices should regularly evaluate their current software and information systems and update them to remain compliant with current regulations.

Implementing the plan

Secure a practice-wide commitment to HIPAA compliance

The privacy regulations require practices to create and implement a privacy compliance plan. To successfully do so, it is important to involve people from several aspects of the practice. These areas should include the dentists or physicians, members of the front desk, billing and collecting, clinical staff (eg, nursing, physician assistants, dental assistants), and administration. Their input can collectively be used to open lines of communication in developing a successful plan.

Designate HIPAA compliance officers and personnel

The compliance personnel consist of the HIPAA privacy and security officers. These people are responsible for leading the compliance efforts. The privacy officer and the security officer can be the same person, especially in small- to mid-sized practices. A large practice may want to outsource one or both positions and should designate someone as the liaison with these positions. Compliance personnel must understand how the practice functions and must have the authority to act to keep the practice compliant, making an administrator, office manager, or the physicians or dentists in the practice good candidates. The HIPAA compliance personnel should be clearly designated in the plan and the practice.

Identify risk areas through a comprehensive information audit

The practice should conduct an organizational evaluation, possibly by an objective third party, and all findings, reports, and actions should be maintained and shared by the compliance personnel, the compliance committee, and the practice board of directors. The following areas should be reviewed: standards and procedures, information system infrastructure, and contracts with business associates. When reviewing standards and procedures, areas where patient confidentiality is at risk need to be identified, and whenever PHI is communicated, patient notice and consent procedures must be in place. Concerning the information system infrastructure, all security concerns should be assessed so that outsiders cannot access the system. Firewalls, passwords, and other security precautions should be considered. The practice should determine which business associates might create or receive PHI, and the appropriate business associate agreements should dictate the nature of the business relationship and how this PHI is used.

Develop and implement practice standards and procedures

One should establish, distribute, and enforce written policies that identify areas of the practice that are at risk. The practice must maintain privacy of PHI as well as security of the information system. The policies should be developed with the compliance personnel and with outside legal counsel, if necessary, and will most likely include the compliance plan, a procedure manual, and other similar items. Some of the minimum areas that need to be addressed within the written policies include proper treatment of PHI, patient notice and consent, staff access to information systems, relationships with other health care providers and business associates (including hospitals, home health agencies, hospices, vendors, pharmaceutical companies, research organizations, and practice advisors). These policies should be reviewed annually and revised when needed.

Conduct appropriate training and education programs

For a compliance plan to be effective, all practice employees should be required to attend mandatory education and training programs on HIPAA compliance. Consider documenting attendance through signed acknowledgments in each employee's personnel file. When creating educational objectives, consider who needs training, the type of training, and when and how frequently the training should occur. The training programs may be external or developed in house, and they should at least cover an overview of HIPAA regulation, identifiable patient record compliance requirements, and a review of the practice HIPAA compliance plan requirements. The following areas should be considered as ongoing areas for training and education: practice policies and procedures regarding privacy practices, security, and data integrity; ongoing compliance efforts including the identification of deficiencies and plans for improvement; and routine updates reflecting changes in the law. If education and training programs are attended outside of the practice, it is recommended that materials from the program be accessible to all practice employees, and that the information learned from the program be shared with all employees.

Establish written agreements with business associates

Practices must have written agreements with business associates so that HIPAA can confirm that the business associates are HIPAA compliant. It is imperative that these agreements are followed. Business associates must abide by the following:

Agree not to use/disclose PHI it receives other than as dictated by contract/law.
Use appropriate safeguards to prevent improper use of PHI.
Report to covered entity any improper/unauthorized use/disclosure of PHI.
Extend compliance obligations to subcontractors.
Make PHI available for inspection, copying, amendment, and accounting.
Make available applicable materials (eg, books, records, information) to the Secretary in the event of a compliance audit of the covered entity.

Return/destroy all applicable PHI at termination of contract, if possible.
Authorize covered entity to terminate contract for material breach.
Agree to right of covered entity to monitor business associate's compliance.
Agree to right of covered entity to cure a breach by business associate.
Use PHI in accordance with applicable law.

The contract must also stipulate under what conditions the business associate may use or disclose PHI. Unless stated otherwise in the contract, business associates may use PHI for management or administration or to provide data aggregation services relating to the health care operations of the covered entity.

Implement procedures to comply with the minimum necessary rule

To ensure that the standards, requirements, and implementation specifications of the minimum necessary rule are met, certain protocols must be developed. The covered entity must decide who in the practice will require PHI access to perform their duties, as well as what type of PHI each employee may need to access. Appropriate conditions should be attached to this access. The practice should then develop protocols for disclosure to ensure that (1) the covered entity creates and implements an evaluation of how to assess a request for PHI; (2) the amount of PHI that is disclosed is limited to the necessary amount for the task; and (3) requests for disclosure of PHI are reviewed along with the protocol on an individual basis.

The exceptions to these protocols are when (1) public officials request PHI, as long as the needed information is the minimum necessary; (2) information is requested by another covered entity, a member of the covered entity's workforce, or a business associate of the covered entity and it is the minimum necessary information needed; and (3) information is requested for research purposes and the requester has followed protocols to request the information.

Responding to violations and developing corrective actions

In regard to suspected HIPAA compliance violations, reports should be documented in conjunction with legal counsel, when appropriate, and investigated by the compliance personnel. If a violation has occurred, the problem needs to be rectified with disciplinary action taken as needed. The HIPAA compliance personnel should document the reported violation, investigation, findings, and any actions taken, and these records should be kept in confidential employee personnel files.

Develop a process to communicate

Compliance personnel should encourage employees to report incidents of noncompliance and should adopt policy that no retaliation will be taken against those reporting the incidents. All efforts should be made to protect the anonymity of those reporting. All complaints should be investigated by the compliance personnel promptly, and legal counsel should be sought if needed. All reports, investigations, findings, actions, questions, and comments should be reported to the board of directors as a written memorandum.

Enforcing disciplinary guidelines

Clear disciplinary guidelines should exist for violations of any law, regulation, requirement, or provision of the HIPAA compliance plan. These guidelines should include a full range from oral warnings to termination of employment. The guidelines should define the actions that may be taken as well as who is responsible for taking the action. The guidelines should apply to all employees of the practice.

HIPAA on marketing the practice

The practice must know under what conditions information is allowed to be sent without authorization while promoting its services. These conditions include the following: (1) marketing materials mailed to patients' homes must identify the practice and the name of the provider who sent them; (2) potential providers must disclose any kind of compensation from any other entity (covered or not) for mailing the solicitation; and (3) if actual marketing material is used, as opposed to broadcast-type or newsletters, the first round of marketing materials must offer an option of declining future solicitations.

There may be a gray area between educating patients generally and advertising services. PHI may be used to identify patients who may benefit from new treatments or services if it is covered in the notice of privacy policies and no authorization is needed. Verbal communication about products or services requires no authorization. No relevant PHI should be disclosed in communications with actual patients unless authorized by the patient.

Develop procedures for patient access to his or her protected health information

Be ready for patient requests to review their medical records and to make amendments if the patient believes the information incorrect. Practices have the right under privacy regulations to include a response to requested patient amendments.

Staff training and policy and procedure book

All office staff must be trained in privacy and security policies, and the records of such training must be maintained. The policies must detail (1) which staff members have access to confidential information, (2) in which circumstances, (3) procedures to be followed when a staff member is terminated, and (4) procedures for identifying and correcting potential problems. The training requirements should be included in a personnel policy manual. In addition, there should be a separate policy manual detailing all privacy and security procedures. If such a policy manual is already in place, it will need to be reviewed to ensure HIPAA requirements are met.

HIPAA in office practice: summary of key points and guidance

The Department of Health and Human Services has released a series of "guidance" recommendations that provide additional explanations for the HIPAA privacy rules as they apply to small practice situations. Responses to issues that have been raised by many providers and the positions of the American Dental Association based on a clarification of HIPAA privacy policy, along with a summary of key HIPAA office practices one must comply with, are as follows [1]:

Dental providers need not restructure their offices (retrofit the office to provide private or soundproof rooms) to comply with HIPAA rules.

Reasonable precautions can be taken to maintain privacy in rooms separated by curtains or screens by speaking in lowered voices.

In small offices, the privacy officer can be the office manager and the training requirement can be met by providing each new employee with a copy of the office privacy policy and documenting that the policies have been reviewed.

Health care providers may discuss a patient's conditions during training rounds in an academic or training institution.

Health care professionals may discuss a patient's condition over the phone with the patient, a provider, or a family member.

The privacy rule does not require encryption of telephone systems.

Soundproofing of rooms is not required.

A dentist may use and disclose PHI for payment purposes.

Patient office visit reminder postcards can be sent through the mail.

A provider only needs to obtain a patient written consent one time (permission to use and disclose PHI to TPO).

Oral communication such as calling out a patient name in a waiting room is permissible.

Sign in sheets for patients at the front desk are permissible as long as the sheet does not contain reasons for the patient's visit.

Patients and non-staff individuals should not be allowed access to any medical records at any place in the office.

Do not post daily patient schedules in plain view.

Do not allow computer screens to be in plain view.

Develop a computer recovery plan in the event of system failure.

Do not leave patient charts around the office.

If the practice maintains a Web site, the notice of privacy practices must be on the Web site.
Distribute a copy of the notice of privacy practices to each patient and receive an acknowledgment of receipt.
Implement security measures to prevent unauthorized access to electronic PHI that is transmitted over electronic communications.

Additional information is available online at multiple Web sites [2–5], with the American Dental Association site being especially helpful.

References

[1] Memo from Dr. James B. Bramson, DDS, Executive Director, HIPAA Privacy Guidance.
[2] Available at: http://www.hhs.gov/ocr/privacy/enforcement.
[3] Available at: http://answers.hhs.gov/cgi-bin/hhs.cfg/php/enduser/stdalp.php.
[4] Available at: http://ada/org/hippa.
[5] Available at: http://aspe.os.dhhs.gov/admnsimp/.

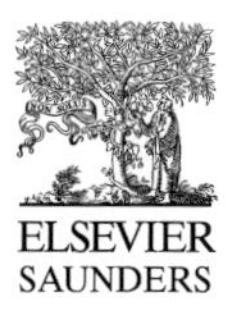

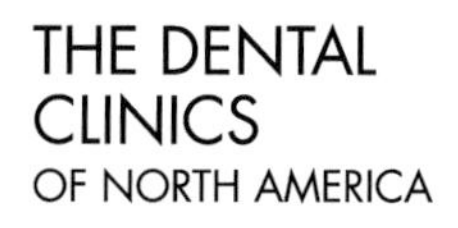

Dent Clin N Am 52 (2008) 683–688

Index

Note: Page numbers of article titles are in **boldface** type.

doi:10.1016/S0011-8532(08)00038-4

D

E

F

G

H

I

J

P

Q

R

S